Because You Care

Other books in the Wisdom & Warnings series

From Divorce Mess to Happiness

Tips From the Quad

Let Them Fly

The Badass Woman

Happily Ever After

Our library of wisdom keeps growing!
Check out the full list anytime at iamjenfort.com/books,
wisdomandwarnings.com or simply scan the QR code.

Because You Care

Your Daily Lifeline Through The Chaos of Caregiving

Jen Fort

From the Wisdom & Warnings®
book series

Disclaimer

The author of *Because You Care* is not a licensed therapist. Because of this, this book is presented solely for educational and entertainment purposes and is not intended to replace the advice of a physician, professional coach, therapist, or other qualified professionals.

This book is available at a discount for bulk purchases in the United States by corporations, institutions and other organizations. For more information, please contact Jen Fort at iamjenfort@gmail.com.

This book was created with the assistance of various resources, including AI as a brainstorming tool to help organize ideas and enhance clarity. However, all insights, concepts, and creative content are entirely the author's.

Cover design by Margaret Cogswell

Edited by Mark Nyman

For Sue—

Thank you for loving my brother with your whole heart. You didn't just care for him... you cared about him. You cheered him on, lifted him up, and made the hard days a bit softer. You balanced care and kindness, setting boundaries when needed, yet giving him the freedom to embrace the simple joys that made him feel like himself... like sneaking out the back door of the hospital for a 'break'.

You are woven into every page of this book because knowing that you loved him so completely reminds me that caregiving, at its core, is about showing up again and again.

With a full heart of deep and never-ending gratitude, this one's for you.

What People Are Saying

"Caregiving pushed me out of my comfort zone and was a very humbling experience. You can make a difference in someone's life and make new friends along the way. Sharing my experiences was very therapeutic for me and I hope it helps other caregivers."

— Donna H.

"This book is a reference tool with nuggets and reminders when the going gets tough."

— Annie R.

Share Your Wisdom!

Wisdom & Warnings consists of nearly 8,000 carefully curated nuggets of wisdom across dozens of topics for life's milestones, ranging from relationships to parents/children to education and career, plus fun topics for living your best life.

Engage with the Wisdom & Warnings community for ongoing encouragement through life's milestones.

www.wisdomandwarnings.com
Facebook: www.facebook.com/wisdomandwarnings/
Instagram: /wisdomandwarnings
Email: hello@wisdomandwarnings.com

My Story

There's something magical about hearing the right words at just the right time—a spark of wisdom that can brighten a day, guide a decision, or even change the course of a life. I've always been drawn to those small but powerful truths. From an early age, I found myself captivated by people's stories; their struggles, triumphs, and the nuggets of wisdom they carried. Every person I met seemed to have something unique to teach me, and I couldn't help but ask: *What's your lesson?*

That curiosity became the seed of a passion I call *Wisdom & Warnings*; a lifelong quest to learn from the experiences of others. Over the years, I turned conversations into a collection of insights. Friends, family, and even strangers at the grocery store shared their advice with me, often without realizing how profound their words were. By the time I looked back, I had gathered over 8,000 pieces of advice; a treasure chest of wisdom just waiting to be shared. But for the longest time, I didn't.

Self-doubt became my shadow. *What if I fail? What if no one cares?* Those questions kept me in a cycle of "someday" and "not yet." I tinkered with the idea for over a decade, hesitating to commit fully. Deep down, though, I couldn't shake the feeling that this treasure wasn't meant to stay hidden. Whenever I thought about shelving the project, a little voice whispered, "Life is too short not to learn from each other." It felt selfish not to share, but fear has a way of making even the brightest ideas feel impossible. That, my friends, is a topic for another time.

Then, life gave me an unexpected push when I lost my job. A moment that felt devastating at first but turned out to be the break I needed. I now had time to reflect, and one thing became crystal clear: it was now or never. Those whispers urging me to share my collection became impossible to ignore. I realized that I didn't need to be perfect or polished; I just needed to start.

So, I took a leap of faith with no formal writing experience and zero understanding of the publishing world. That leap became the *365 Days of Wisdom & Warnings* book series. Along the way, I've made mistakes, learned lessons, and celebrated every small victory. More than anything, I've realized that when you listen to the quiet whispers of your heart, you're led to something greater than fear: purpose.

If this journey has taught me anything, it's that the world needs what only you can offer. You might feel unqualified or unsure, but someone out there is waiting for what you have to give. My wish for you is this: trust those quiet whispers, silence the doubts; whether they're yours or someone else's—and chase what sets your soul on fire. Your passion could be the light that sparks someone else's journey. And isn't that the real magic?

I'll be cheering you on,

Jen

Introduction

Welcome to this book, and a quiet space where you can breathe, even for a moment. *Because You Care* was created with the unexpected caregiver in mind, because you are the one holding so much together while often feeling like you're coming apart.

Whether you're just stepping into caregiving or have been walking this path for years, the encouragement was curated with you in mind. This book won't sugarcoat the hard stuff, and it won't pretend to have all the answers. What it *will* do is walk beside you, offering one small bit of support a day to help lighten your emotional load, soothe your tired spirit, and remind you: you are not alone.

Inside these pages, you'll find practical tips, heartfelt truths, and gentle nudges—all drawn from real people who've walked this caregiving road themselves. They've stumbled, adapted, loved fiercely, and generously shared what helped them through. Some days, the wisdom here will lift your spirits. Other days, it'll offer a laugh, a fresh perspective, or a gentle reminder that you matter too. You'll find encouragement to set boundaries, take a breath, ask for help, and release the pressure to do it all perfectly. This isn't polished advice from a podium—it's real talk from the trenches, offered with love, honesty, and hope.

Let this be your daily companion. A reminder that strength isn't about never breaking, it's about showing up with compassion, even on the days you feel exhausted.

You are doing something extraordinary. One day at a time.

Day 1

Trust your intuition, even if it seems bizarre.

There will be times when your gut speaks louder than any book or expert. And yes, sometimes it whispers ideas that feel strange or unconventional. But that voice inside? It's rooted in love, your own personal lived experience, and your unique connection to the person you're caring for. Intuition is not a magical power; it's a finely tuned instrument built over time. Don't dismiss it just because it doesn't follow a plan or prescription. Some of the most impactful decisions you'll ever make will be based on what "just felt right." Trust that. Your intuition isn't weird, it's wise. Listen closely. It won't steer you wrong.

Day 2

*It's not the load that breaks you;
it's the way you carry it.*

Caregiving comes with a heavy bag of responsibilities, but how you shoulder that weight makes all the difference. Are you balancing it with rest, support, and moments of joy? Or dragging it solo with guilt and self-neglect stuffed in the side pockets? The load itself may not change, but you can. Ask for help. Adjust expectations. Put down perfectionism because it's heavier than it looks. Redistribute the emotional weight so it doesn't all fall on your shoulders. You're not weak for feeling overwhelmed; you're resourceful for changing the way you carry the hard stuff.

Day 3

*Listen to people who encourage you to do what
you know is right in your heart.*

When you're stretched thin, everyone suddenly has an opinion about what you should do. But caregiving isn't a one-size-fits-all journey. It's deeply personal. The voices that matter most are the ones that remind you to trust yourself, the ones who encourage you to listen to that quiet knowing inside your own heart. You're closer to the situation than anyone else, and you carry wisdom even when you feel unsure. Take advice with a grain of salt and protect your right to choose what feels best for you and your loved one. Trust yourself. You are doing sacred, hard work, and no one knows your path better than you do.

Day 4

No one said it would be easy.

There's no sugarcoating it... **this road is hard.** Some days will stretch your patience, drain your energy, and weigh heavily on your heart. I won't tell you it's always going to feel worth it in the moment, because some days it just won't. But here's what I *can* tell you: the love you give, the quiet sacrifices, the way you keep showing up—it all matters more than you realize. Even when you're running on empty, you're making a difference in someone's life. So, take a breath and keep going. One day, you'll look back and realize just how much strength and beauty were woven into those toughest moments.

Day 5

You might not see it, but the routines you create have the most profound impact.

You're not expected to be a miracle worker. But every time you create a rhythm, consistent routine, a comforting space, or a plan they can rely on, you are giving the gift of peace. That's no small thing. It lowers anxiety, builds trust, and makes the hard days more bearable. Predictability says, "You're safe. You're cared for. We've got this." Your impact makes a positive difference, even if the illness doesn't change. Don't discount the power of steady love. Your behind-the-scenes efforts are the framework holding everything together.

Day 6

Caring for another person is hard work; some days are simply a little less hard.

You won't get a trophy. You might not even get a thank-you. But please know this: showing up every day, in big and small ways, is a quiet kind of heroism. Some days you'll feel strong. Others? Not so much. But you're still doing it. And that's remarkable. Not perfect. Not polished. But real. You're making a difference, even during the days you doubt it. So, before you crash into bed tonight, remind yourself: "I did my best with what I had." That matters. You matter. Keep going. And if today was messy? Fantastic. You still showed up. That's everything.

Day 7

Act on goals, not emotions.

Caregiving stirs up a lot of emotions: frustration, guilt, sadness, even bursts of anger. Those feelings are real and valid, but they don't always make the best compass. When life gets stormy, try to anchor yourself to your goals, not your emotions. What matters most today? Maybe it's getting your loved one to that appointment, or perhaps it's carving out twenty minutes of quiet for yourself. Let your deeper intentions, not your moment-to-moment feelings, guide your next step. Emotions will ebb and flow, but your goals are the steady ground you can keep returning to. One small, purposeful step at a time is enough.

Day 8

People might not understand your journey and that's okay.

Caregiving can feel isolating, not because you're alone, but because few people truly understand the scope. Some people will question your choices, offer shallow advice, or disappear totally. That's okay. Your journey wasn't assigned to anyone else; it was given to you for reasons that may never be fully visible from the outside. You don't need validation from anyone. You need strength, grace, and the occasional deep breath. Keep walking along your path, even if others don't see the road beneath your feet. Their understanding isn't required for your steps to be right. This journey is personal and powerful.

Day 9

You can do anything, but not everything.

Yes, you're strong. Yes, you're capable. But even superheroes need backup. Just because you can do something doesn't mean you should do it all. Let go of the pressure to manage every detail, meet every need, fix every problem. Delegate. Rest. Prioritize. You are not failing, you're human. And humans have limits. Honor them. Protect your peace. Choose what matters most and give yourself grace for what falls through the cracks. The world doesn't need you to do everything. It needs you to last.

Day 10

Listen to what doctors say, as well as what they don't say.

When you're in the room with a doctor, pay attention not just to the words they speak, but also to the ones they *don't*. Sometimes what's missing says as much as what's shared. A pause, a vague answer, or a change in tone can all be quiet signals worth noticing. Ask questions. Trust your gut. You know your loved one best, and your role includes reading between the lines. Listening with both ears and trusting your instincts can help you advocate more effectively, catch what others might miss, and make decisions with deeper understanding.

Day 11

*Be ready for drastic and surprising changes
in your friendships.*

Caregiving changes absolutely everything in your life, not just your routines. It can profoundly affect your relationships. Some friends will quietly disappear, unsure of how to show up or simply unwilling to. That's a mix of hurt and disappointment. But others will step forward, sometimes unexpectedly, offering kindness, presence, and unwavering support. This season reveals who's here for the highlight reel and who's willing to stay for the bloopers. Mourn the losses but celebrate the gains. The friendships that survive or begin during this time are forged in something real and lasting. Let the shifting sands settle. You may end up with fewer friends, but they'll be truer and stronger.

Day 12

There is freedom in saying "No."

"No" is not a rejection; it's a declaration of value. Every time you say no to something that drains you, you're saying yes to your health, your peace, and your priorities. You're not being rude. You're being real. Caregivers often feel pressure to be everything to everyone. But you're allowed to draw a line. You don't have to explain or apologize. "No" can be loving, protective, and wise. Practice saying "No" often, because you'll make space for what matters, and be able to put behind what doesn't

Day 13

*If you have a child with disabilities, you can
involve their siblings in simple tasks.*

Kids want to help. Involving siblings in simple, age-appropriate caregiving tasks for their disabled sibling helps them feel connected, capable, and included. Let them press play on the movie. Hand over a book to read out loud. Ask for help fetching a toy or adjusting a pillow. These little tasks build empathy without creating resentment. Just be careful not to turn them into mini caregivers. This is about connection, not delegation. Keep it light. Praise their help. Let them contribute without pressure. When done right, you're not just managing care, you're strengthening the bond between siblings in a way that lasts beyond the hard days.

Day 14

*The hardest decisions are usually the most impactful;
don't stick your head in the sand.*

Hard decisions are the uninvited guests of caregiving—they barge in, make you uncomfortable, and linger way too long. But they often carry the power to change things for the better. Whether it's setting boundaries, saying no, or choosing a new direction for care, these decisions aren't easy, but they're often necessary. Avoiding them only intensifies your stress and prolongs the pain. Face these decisions with clarity, compassion, and backup if needed. You don't have to be fearless, just courageous. Hard choices aren't a sign of failure; they're a sign you're stepping up. They often become turning points in a journey that needs a shift.

Day 15

Don't play the "What If" game.

"What if I had done it differently?" "What if I make the wrong call?" That loop in your mind is endless, exhausting, and let's face it, totally unfair to yourself. You're making decisions in real time, with limited information and a heart full of love. You don't need to rewrite the past or fear the future... the future hasn't arrived yet. Stay rooted in what is. Focus on what you can do, not what you could have. The What If game steals peace, second-guesses your instincts, and serves no reward. Replace it with "What's next?" or "What's needed now?" That's where your power lives. Play that game instead.

Day 16

Don't wait to tackle difficult tasks until you're tired.

Difficult tasks have a sneaky way of growing fangs the longer you wait. And if you save them for when you're running on fumes, they'll only feel heavier. Instead, hit them while your brain still has battery life. Early in the day, after rest, or post-coffee, whenever you feel most mentally alert. You'll think clearly, act faster, and feel more accomplished afterward. Don't let dread drag all day. Cross it off early, reclaim your mental space, and give your future self a high five. Tackling hard things when you're fresh turns mountains into molehills. Bonus: you might even have time for a nap.

Day 17

You must come to terms with the changes and learn to accept your loved one as they are now.

Change in caregiving can feel like a slow heartbreak; watching someone you love shift from who they were to who they are now. It's natural to want things to stay the same, to hold on to the "before," but resisting the changes only deepens the pain. Acceptance doesn't mean you like it or that it's easy; it means you're choosing to meet this moment as it is, not as you wish it were. When you can do that, you create space for grace, patience, and even small joys in the "now." It's a tender kind of strength, but one that will carry you through.

Day 18

Most caregivers don't plan it; they simply step in when life calls, often without warning.

You didn't plan this. You weren't handed a rulebook or given time to prepare. One moment you were helping out... and then suddenly, you were the caregiver. It happens gradually, and then all at once. Know this: you're not alone. Many people walk into caregiving by accident, not by choice, but by necessity. That doesn't make you less qualified; it makes you human. You're learning on the fly, adapting daily, and doing your best with what you've got. It's okay to feel unready. No one feels fully ready. You stepped in because you care—and that makes all the difference.

Day 19

Doctors don't always have the answers.

Doctors are incredibly knowledgeable, but they're not magicians. Sometimes, even with all their training and tests, there aren't clear answers. That can be frustrating, and scary, especially when you're desperate for certainty. But medicine is part science, part mystery, and not every outcome comes with a guarantee. It's okay to feel uneasy in that gray space. Just remember, not having all the answers doesn't mean no one cares or nothing can be done. It means decisions may come down to trust, instincts, and what feels right for your loved one and your family.

Day 20

You must hold sacred time with other people you love.

Caregiving can easily consume every ounce of your time and energy, but you can't let it crowd out your other relationships. The people you love, such as your partner, kids, and friends, are part of what keeps you grounded and whole. Hold that time sacred, even if it's just a quick coffee, a phone call, or a quiet dinner without interruptions. Those moments refill your heart and remind you that your world is bigger than caregiving. Nurturing those connections isn't selfish, it's essential. It keeps you human, balanced, and better able to show up for the one you're caring for.

Day 21

Keep a sense of humor.

Laughter may not refill prescriptions or schedule appointments, but it will save your sanity. Caregiving brings absurd, awkward, and downright ridiculous moments; laugh at them. Spilled meds, uncomfortable silences, or conversations with doctors that sound like a foreign language? Giggle. Snort. Scream into your pillow if needed. Oh, and throw in a bit of sarcasm, that helps me! Humor doesn't diminish the seriousness of what you're doing; it enables you to survive it. A well-timed joke can soften a hard day, and sometimes laughing is the most rational response. Keep your sense of humor close; it's the cheapest therapy around. You're already carrying enough; don't forget to lighten it with a bit of joy.

Day 22

Stay connected to the world outside of caregiving.

Isolation often slips in slowly, unnoticed, until one day you realize how long it's been since you had a real conversation that wasn't about medications or appointments. That's why staying connected to the outside world must be intentional. Even a quick text, a short call, or a coffee with a friend can breathe life back into your day. You don't have to carry this alone, and you're not meant to. Let connection be a lifeline; it keeps your world bigger than caregiving and reminds you that you still matter, too.

Day 23

Choose your battles wisely.

Caregiving is a full-time job, and guess what? You don't have the energy to fight every battle. Not every hill is worth dying on. Some things deserve your effort, and others deserve a shrug and a snack. Is this a moment to stand firm, or is it one you can release with grace? Ask yourself: Will this matter tomorrow? Next week? In a year? If not, let it go. Save your strength for what truly matters; health, peace, love, and chocolate. You've got too much on your plate to waste time on every disagreement. Choose wisely. You're a caregiver, not a gladiator.

Day 24

"If you're going through Hell, keep going."
— Winston Churchill

When caregiving feels like an endless tunnel of exhaustion and uncertainty, the most important thing you can do is to *keep going.* This isn't where you're meant to stay; it's just where you are right now. Think of it like going to the gym: if you stop showing up, starting again feels ten times harder. Every muscle aches, and it takes all your willpower to get moving. But if you keep going, even if you need to slow down for a day or two, your strength builds, your stamina grows, and your body starts to thank you. Caregiving is no different. Forward is still forward, even if it's a shuffle. Don't let the challenging moments convince you to quit. You're not stuck; you're strengthening.

Day 25

Pretending to be strong is exhausting.

Real strength doesn't come from plastered smiles or pretending everything's fine when you're unraveling. Caregiving is hard, and no amount of emotional duct tape will hold forever. Allow yourself a good cry when you need to; it's not a sign of weakness, it's a release. Let life hit you, move through you, and build you. Tears aren't the opposite of strength; they're proof of it. You're letting yourself feel and still choosing to carry on. That's the real muscle. So, drop the performance. Be messy, honest, and human. True strength is born in the spaces where you stop faking it and start feeling it.

Day 26

You may not want to cut ties with a negative friend, but you MUST create firm boundaries and limit your time with them.

Protecting your peace is not selfish; it's survival. You're already carrying a heavy load; don't let draining people pile more on. Maybe it's a friend who minimizes your role, or someone who makes everything about themselves. You don't have to cut them out completely, but you do have to draw the line. Limit interactions, be honest, and set expectations. You don't owe anyone unlimited access to your energy. Your focus is on caregiving, healing, and self-care. And that's more than enough. Boundaries aren't rejection; they're protection. And you, dear one, are worth protecting.

Day 27

If you keep your stress held inside, at some point you will boil over.

Bottled-up stress has a funny way of showing up at the worst time—in traffic, in tears, or a loud outburst over something small. You need a pressure valve. Someone who gets it. Someone who lets you say, "This sucks," without judgment. It could be a friend, a support group, a therapist, or even a stranger on a helpline. Talk. Cry. Laugh about the absurd stuff. Caregiving is too heavy to carry silently. You're allowed to offload. You're allowed to vent. Find people who listen without fixing. You don't need perfect advice; you need safe ears so you can release before you explode.

Day 28

A good therapist can be life-changing.

A therapist can be a powerful support, but finding the right one is key. It's okay (and wise) to speak with a few before committing. You need someone who gets you, listens without judgment, and creates a space where you can breathe. Once you choose, give it a solid two months. If, after that, you still don't feel fully supported or understood, don't settle... switch. Therapy isn't one-size-fits-all, and you deserve a fit that feels right. The right therapist won't just listen; they'll help you carry what feels too heavy. Continue searching until you find the kind of support you're looking for. It's totally worth it.

Day 29

Make sure you have three friends:
The Comedian, The Rock, and The Resource.

Caregiving requires a dream team, and not just of doctors and aides. You need three kinds of friends: The Comedian, who reminds you to laugh when you'd rather cry; The Rock, who stands steady when you wobble; and The Resource, who knows all the hacks, contacts, and calming tea blends. One lifts your spirit, one holds your hand, and one hands you the map. Each plays a vital role. Don't try to do it all alone; build your support squad. These aren't just friends; they're lifelines. Find them, thank them, and keep them close.

Day 30

When hearing advice, just nod your head,
then do what feels right.

Caregiving attracts advice like a porch light attracts moths—constant, fluttering, and occasionally annoying. Smile, nod, and graciously accept the insight... then go do what aligns with your instincts and situation. Most advice is given with love, but only you know the whole picture. What works for one family may be a disaster for yours. So, smile and thank the advice-givers, file away the helpful nuggets, and toss the rest like mismatched socks. Your path requires courage, not consensus. You're allowed to trust your gut, even if it disagrees with Aunt Marge or Dr. Google.

Day 31

Give good news quick... bad news quicker.

When it comes to caregiving communication, don't play emotional hide-and-seek. Share the good stuff with joy and speed; celebrate wins, no matter how small. But also, don't delay the tough conversations. Bad news doesn't age well; it festers. Being direct and timely isn't cruel, it's respectful. It provides people with space to process, adapt, and support one another. You're not a news anchor, but many are looking to you for the truth. Deliver it with kindness, but don't sugarcoat it into confusion. Whether it's progress or a setback, clarity is a gift. Be honest, be swift, and be compassionate. It builds trust, and that trust goes a long way.

Day 32

Therapy brings hard truths—don't run.
Facing them is where the healing begins.

Therapy can be a lifeline for caregivers, but it's not always easy. Sometimes it brings up hard truths you've been too busy or too tired to face: the resentment, the guilt, or the grief you've tucked away to keep going. Don't run from those feelings. Naming them doesn't make you a bad caregiver; it makes you an honest one. Working through those truths is how you begin to heal, even while you're still in the thick of it. You're carrying a lot. Therapy helps you unpack some of it, so the weight isn't all on you. Let that be part of your care, too.

Day 33

Simplify choices to make life easier for everyone.

Decision fatigue is a real thing, especially when it comes to caregiving. The brain can only make so many choices before it begins to short-circuit. Reduce the mental clutter where you can: meal plans, labeled drawers, routines, or pre-filled forms. Let your loved one choose between two options instead of open-ended questions. Set up systems that repeat. Fewer choices = fewer stress points. Simplification isn't laziness, it's wisdom. It frees your brain for what matters most: compassion, connection, and calmness. Life is already complicated. Give yourself and those you love the gift of simplicity.

Day 34

Don't sweat the things you cannot control,
but control the things you can.

Control is a slippery thing, especially when caregiving throws curveballs faster than you can duck. You can't fix every moment, but you can shape your response. Focus on the things within reach: your attitude, your boundaries, your rest, your breath. Let the rest go; yes, even if it drives you bonkers. Worrying over what you can't control is like trying to staple water. Instead, redirect your energy toward what's manageable. You'll feel more grounded and less like you're spinning in circles. Serenity isn't passive; it's strategic. Tighten the grip where it matters. Loosen it where it doesn't. You've got this—one deep breath at a time.

Day 35

It takes a village to care for someone.

You may feel like you have to carry everything yourself, but caregiving is not meant to be a solo sport. Whether it's family, friends, neighbors, or professionals, build your village. Communicate. Delegate. Trust others to step in. Each person brings a different gift to the circle: patience, humor, cooking, and logistics. Use them all. Asking for help isn't weakness, it's wisdom. You're not proving your strength by burning out. You're proving your love by letting it be sustainable. The best care doesn't come from one exhausted person; it comes from a whole team showing up together.

Day 36

Hospice is so much more than end-of-life care.

Hospice isn't just about dying; it's about living well in the time that remains. It brings comfort, dignity, and support—not just to the person in care, but to the entire family. Nurses, social workers, chaplains, and aides collaborate to alleviate physical pain and emotional stress. Many families say, "I wish we'd called sooner." It's not giving up; it's leaning into peace. Hospice services are often covered by insurance as well. Don't let the word scare you. Learn what it means. Hospice walks alongside you at one of life's hardest chapters—and makes sure you don't walk it alone.

Day 37

Humor can be a wonderful stress reliever.

Sometimes the only thing left to do is laugh. When caregiving gets absurd, exhausting, or just plain surreal, humor can pull you back from the edge. Find the funny, even if it's dark or inappropriate. Giggle at the mismatched socks, the third spilled coffee, or the fact that you're crying and laughing at the same time. Humor is medicine for the soul, and often the quickest way to reconnect with yourself and your loved one. Watch a funny show. Swap ridiculous stories with a friend. Release the pressure valve. You don't have to be serious all the time. Laugh. Loudly. Often.

Day 38

It doesn't always get better; it gets different.

People mean well when they say, "It'll get better." But let's be honest—sometimes it doesn't. What it gets is different. You adjust. You develop new rhythms. The pain doesn't disappear, but it loses its sharp edges. The situation may not change drastically, but you do. That's not settling—it's evolving. The hard days still exist, but so do pockets of grace, new strengths, and unexpected moments of joy. Let go of waiting for things to "go back to normal." Instead, create a new normal that includes space for healing, laughter, and growth. Different doesn't mean worse; it can mean deeper. More human. More real.

Day 39

*Having separate accounts for your money and
the person you care for can be essential.*

Love and finances are a tricky mix. For everyone's protection (including yours), it's wise to keep personal and caregiving finances separate. It helps avoid confusion, keeps tax time simpler, and ensures accountability. If others ever step in to help, keep clear records to prevent misunderstandings. It's not about distrust; it's about transparency. Create a basic system. Track what's spent, what's reimbursed, and what belongs to whom. Down the road, this kind of organization can save you from emotional and legal headaches. You're not being distant, you're being responsible. Love with your heart but lead with your head. Separate accounts help you do both.

Day 40

*You will grieve in small doses—just don't let it
spill onto the one you're caring for.*

Grief doesn't wait for the final goodbye; it shows up in small doses, day by day. You may mourn the changes, the losses, and the life that once was. That's normal, and it's human. But try not to let that grief spill over in front of the person you're caring for. They're carrying their own emotional weight, and your calm presence can be a source of comfort. Find your own space to grieve; whether that includes holding quiet moments, talking to trusted friends, keeping a journal, or seeing a therapist. You *need* those outlets. Remember to protect your loved one's space while honoring your own feelings. Both can coexist with care and with grace.

Day 41

Know that it's OK to laugh, cry, and anything in between.

Caregiving isn't all tears or all triumph; it's the wild in-between. One minute you're crying in the car, the next you're laughing at an absurd moment involving misplaced dentures and a barking Alexa. Emotions don't arrive in a single file, they come in waves, sometimes crashing into each other. That's not dysfunction, that's reality. Allow yourself to experience the full spectrum without judgment. This journey is deeply human, and so are you. Laugh when it's funny, cry when it's hard, and dance like no one's watching; especially when they're watching. You're not a robot. Feel the feelings; that's how healing happens.

Day 42

Learn how others in a similar situation have coped.

You're not alone; even if it feels that way. Other caregivers have walked this path, stubbed their toes on the same rocks, and found clever ways around emotional potholes. Tap into that wisdom. Join a support group, read their stories, and ask questions. You don't have to reinvent the caregiving wheel—someone else has already patched the tire. Learning from others isn't a weakness; it's a strategy. It brings relief, perspective, and a sense of community. And let's be honest, some of the best coping tips come from those who've cried in their car, laughed during hospice visits, and still managed to make dinner. You don't have to do this alone. Learn from your people.

Day 43

Choosing a care facility can take months; give yourself the time to get it right.

Choosing a care facility, whether it's adult daycare, respite care, or long-term placement, isn't something to rush. It may take weeks or even months to find the right fit, and that's okay. You're not just picking a building, you're trusting people with someone you love. Pay attention to the staff: are they kind, patient, and transparent? Do they answer your questions clearly and allow you to tour freely? If you feel rushed, dismissed, or restricted from seeing certain areas, consider it a red flag. Trust your inner voice. The right place will welcome your curiosity and understand how big this decision really is. Take your time. Your loved one and you deserve that.

Day 44

Make sure you have a special 'thing' with the other members of your family.

Caregiving can consume your time, but don't let it swallow your relationships. Set aside one special tradition with each family member, something simple, doable, and just for the two of you. An ice cream run. A five-minute dance party. A Sunday crossword. These moments become sacred. They remind your family that they matter outside the caregiving bubble. Protect those rituals and guard that space. It doesn't have to be fancy; it just has to be consistent. Your relationships also need room to grow. And those little traditions? They're lifelines disguised as joy. Hold onto them.

Day 45

Life is a balance of holding on and letting go.

Caregiving is the constant dance of clinging and releasing. You hold on to memories, routines, dignity, and yet you're constantly letting go of expectations, control, and even parts of yourself. Both actions are sacred. The strength lies not in choosing one over the other, but in knowing when to use each. Some days, you'll fiercely protect what matters most. Other days, you'll exhale and release what's too heavy to carry. This balance isn't a weakness; it's wisdom. You are strong enough to hold on with love and brave enough to let go with grace. And in the middle is where peace begins to grow.

Day 46

If you think you must do it all, you are mistaken.

You don't have to be everything to everyone. That belief is a fast track to burnout. Yes, you're strong. Yes, you're resourceful. But you are not invincible. You're human, and you deserve rest, help, and compassion too. The dishes can wait. The texts can go unanswered. The world won't crumble if you say "no" or ask for help. Let go of the guilt. Caregiving doesn't require martyrdom; it requires sustainability. Save your energy for what truly matters and let the rest go. You are already doing so much. Permit yourself what you'd give a friend: moments to stop, breathe, and be.

Day 47

*What seems logical to you might not feel logical
to the one you're caring for.*

The way you see a situation may be completely different from how your loved one experiences it. Illness, memory challenges, or a loss of independence can shift their perspective, making your "obvious" solution feel confusing or even upsetting to them. Instead of pushing to be understood, try leaning into empathy and curiosity. What matters most is not who's right. Rather, it's about finding a path that's supportive and respectful. Sometimes the most loving choice is to let go of logic and simply meet them where they are.

Day 48

*Some days, everything is going your way; other
days, you feel like your world is crumbling.*

There are days when the stars align; appointments are kept, meds are taken, and you even get to drink your coffee while it's still hot. Then there are days when everything seems to unravel at once. Breathe. These moments aren't the end; they're just the messy middle. You're allowed to feel overwhelmed, but don't dwell there. Push through, even if your pace slows to a crawl. One small step is still forward motion. On the hard days, remind yourself: this too shall pass. Maybe like a kidney stone, but it will pass. Hang in there. Your strength is showing, even when you're shaking.

Day 49

Words are not always necessary.

Care often goes far beyond conversation. Sometimes, love is communicated through a glance, a touch, or the silent language of being fully present. You don't need perfect words to bring peace. You need presence. Sit quietly. Notice their eyes. Respond to their gestures. Even when they can't speak, they are still telling you something. Connection doesn't require dialogue; it needs attention. And sometimes, the most meaningful moments come without a single word. Let your heart be the translator. Love has a way of speaking for itself.

Day 50

Social workers, service providers, healthcare professionals, and lawyers can help you learn about services and plans for the future.

You don't have to figure everything out alone. There's a whole ecosystem of professionals who've walked beside other caregivers and know the ropes. A social worker can help you access programs, respite care, or financial support. A lawyer can guide you through legal documents. Healthcare providers can direct you to specialists. Don't wait for crisis mode; ask now. Be proactive. Build your team. Because while love is your fuel, knowledge is your map. And in caregiving, both are essential. Help is out there. Don't be afraid to take it.

Day 51

It's okay not to know everything!!

Spoiler alert: no one has it all figured out. Caregiving doesn't come with a manual—and even if it did, the pages would probably be stuck together with tears and coffee. Not knowing something doesn't make you unqualified; it makes you human. Ask questions, Google shamelessly, and lean on those who've walked this road before. You're not weak for admitting you need help; you're wise for knowing you can't go it alone. Release the pressure to be perfect. You are learning, adjusting, and showing up every day; and that counts. Give yourself grace because you're doing far better than you think. Seriously.

Day 52

Take everyone's advice with a grain of salt.

Advice is everywhere: blogs, books (even this one), and strangers in the doctor's office waiting room. Everyone's got an opinion, especially when they're not the ones in the trenches. But caregiving isn't one-size-fits-all. What worked beautifully for someone else might be a dumpster fire in your world. So, listen politely, thank them for their insight, then run it through your own filter. Keep what resonates. Toss the rest. You are the expert in your own experience, and your intuition matters more than someone else's opinion. Advice is seasoning, not the main dish. Sprinkle it wisely. And when in doubt, trust your gut. It's got excellent taste.

Day 53

Be patient and gentle with an angry person.

Anger is often grief dressed in armor. The person you care for may lash out, not because of you, but because of their loss of independence, clarity, and control. It's not personal, though it sure can feel that way. Meet their fire with patience. Not because you're a doormat, but because you're wise enough to see the pain beneath the rage. Stay grounded. Set healthy boundaries, but also respond with gentleness when possible. Your calm can be the mirror that reflects their humanity. It's not easy, but it's powerful. Patience isn't weakness; it's love wearing armor of its own.

Day 54

Starting each day with a positive quote or mantra sets the tone for the remainder of the day.

Before the emails, alarms, and responsibilities crash in, take one minute to center yourself. Read a quote, whisper a mantra, or say something kind to yourself in the mirror. This tiny ritual can shift your entire mindset. You're not just reacting; you're choosing how to begin. Try, "I am doing the best I can," or "Peace is my priority today." Write it down. Tape it to your fridge. Let it anchor you when the chaos hits. The day may still be messy but let your first thought be one of hope.

Day 55

*Schedule fun activities on days when your loved one
is not feeling the side effects of treatment.*

Some days, you plan everything, and nothing goes as planned. But when energy allows, having something to look forward to, no matter how small, can make all the difference. Maybe it's a picnic, a movie night, or just sitting in the sun. Look for windows of good energy and fill them with light moments. Planning can feel daunting when life is so unpredictable, but even tentative plans give hope, and hope is powerful. You're not just managing care, you're making space for joy, even five minutes of it. That counts.

Day 56

*If a support group is focused on negativity and
competition, find a new group.*

Support should feel like a warm hug, not a competition. If your group is more about venting than growing, or if you walk away feeling worse, trust your gut; it's not your place. The right tribe uplifts, shares honestly, and holds space for both tears and triumphs. Whether in-person or online, find your people. The ones who offer wisdom without judgment, humor without sarcasm, and encouragement without pity. You deserve support that fills your cup, not drains it. Your energy is sacred. Share it where it grows.

Day 57

Lack of self-care will affect your attention to detail.

When you're running on empty, the little things start to slip, and in caregiving, those details matter. Skipping meals, losing sleep, or ignoring your own needs can cloud your focus, making it easier to miss medication times, overlook changes in behavior, or forget small but important tasks. It's not about being perfect, it's about being present, and you can't do that if you're running on fumes. Taking care of yourself sharpens your mind and steadies your energy, allowing you to show up fully for yourself and those you care for. Think of self-care not as a luxury, but as maintenance for the most important tool you have: *you.*

Day 58

Family can help you through good times and bad.
This applies to friends who are also family.

When life turns sideways, you quickly discover who your true friends are. Sometimes it's family by blood; other times, it's the friend who shows up with soup, sarcasm, or just silence. Lean into the ones who bring peace, not pressure. These are the folks who remind you who you are, even when you forget. They know your quirks, yet they still choose to stay. Let them in. Let them help. You don't need to be a lone ranger with a to-do list. Whether it's your cousin, neighbor, or best friend since third grade, your circle matters. Let your village love and support you.

Day 59

Happiness can be found in the darkest of times.

Dark moments will visit, such as grief, fatigue, fear, but that doesn't mean joy is gone for good. Sometimes it's hiding, waiting for you to switch your focus. Turning on the light can be as simple as noticing a good cup of coffee, a shared laugh, or a breath of fresh air. You don't have to deny the darkness to acknowledge the light. They can exist together. Choose to seek out small moments of gladness. It won't fix everything, but it will warm your spirit. You don't need blinding brightness; just a flicker of hope. That's how you make your way through the shadows.

Day 60

When memory fails, emotions remain.

When memory begins to fade, it's the emotions that stay behind. A person with dementia may not recall the exact day, the location, or even the names, but they'll remember how they *felt*. They may forget which beach you visited, but they'll remember the joy of the waves or the warmth of the sun. Trying to force specifics can lead to frustration for both of you. Instead, focus on the feelings. Create moments that feel peaceful, joyful, or safe. Because in the end, it's not the details that last; it's the emotional imprint you leave behind. That's what lingers. That's what matters.

Day 61

*Realize that people may not offer help because
they don't know how to ask.*

It's not that people don't care, it's that they're unsure how to step in. They worry about saying the wrong thing or interrupting at an inopportune moment. Instead of offering specifics, they remain silent. Don't take it personally. If someone says, "Let me know if I can help," that's your cue: be direct: "Yes, can you sit with Mom for two hours Friday?" or "A hot meal next week would be a gift." Give them something concrete. Most people want to help—they just need guidance. Don't be shy about handing them the playbook. You don't have to do it alone.

Day 62

It can be difficult to envision the unknown.

When you're in the thick of caregiving, the future can feel like a foggy road—no clear signs and no guaranteed outcomes. That uncertainty can be unsettling. We humans crave direction, clarity, and a plan. But sometimes the path ahead isn't mapped yet because you're still building it. That's okay! It's not your job to predict every twist and turn. It's your job to keep showing up, one step at a time. Trust that clarity will come, even if it's not here yet. Let hope be your flashlight. You may not see far ahead, but you can see enough to keep going.

Day 63

Create an online volunteer care calendar.

You don't have to carry it all; especially when technology can help. Use free online tools like Lotsa Helping Hands or CaringBridge to set up a care calendar. It's an easy way for friends, family, and neighbors to help without the endless, "Let me know if you need anything" back-and-forth. Want someone to bring dinner? Watch your loved one while you nap? Pick up meds? Put it on the calendar. Let people sign up and show up. It makes support practical, organized, and consistent, and it removes the awkwardness of asking. Caregiving is a team sport. Let tech be your assistant coach.

Day 64

Have some healthy to-go meal options readily available so you care for yourself, even when busy.

Caregivers often skip meals, as if it were a sport. But you can't pour from an empty stomach. Stock up on easy, nutritious options: protein bars, hard-boiled eggs, fruit, yogurt, even peanut butter sandwiches. The goal isn't gourmet food; it's practical food. Pre-cut veggies and deli wraps are a healthier alternative to fast food or skipping dinner altogether. Throw a snack in your bag every time you leave the house. Hydration matters too, so keep water nearby. You wouldn't let your loved one go without meals—don't do it to yourself. You're not being selfish by eating, you're being smart.

Day 65

Silliness helps relieve stress.

Sure, you're dealing with serious things, but that doesn't mean you have to be serious all the time. Goofy moments are lifesavers. A funny face, a ridiculous dance move, a poorly timed pun are not just comic relief; they're survival tactics. Laughter serves as a pressure valve, releasing tension and giving your nervous system a break. Let yourself giggle. Let your loved one be silly. Even a shared smile can shift the whole atmosphere. Don't underestimate humor's healing power. Life may be heavy, but your spirit doesn't have to be. When in doubt, embrace the silly. It's sanity in disguise.

Day 66

There are programs and ways to become a paid caregiver for a loved one.

Caring for a loved one can take a significant financial toll, but you may have options available. In many states, programs are available that allow family caregivers to receive compensation for their time and effort. These aren't charity; they're recognition that what you're doing is work. Explore resources at AARP.org, your local Department of Aging, or Medicaid waiver programs. Ask questions and advocate for yourself. Don't assume help isn't available. Getting paid doesn't change your love; it supports your ability to keep showing up with energy and dignity. You deserve to be cared for, too. And that includes financial peace of mind.

Day 67

*Too much information can lead to
feeling overwhelmed.*

Information can be helpful, but too much of it can leave you feeling anxious, overwhelmed, and stuck in worst-case scenarios. Between the internet, WebMD, books, doctors, and well-meaning friends, it's easy to drown in facts and forecasts. Sometimes, the best thing you can do is step back and focus on today. You already see the changes and feel the shifts. You don't need to memorize every symptom or worry about what might happen six months from now, like forgetting how to smile. Take it one day, one moment, at a time. Trust what you see and know. The rest can wait.

Day 68

*Failing to prioritize self-care can lead
to a downward spiral.*

Skipping self-care isn't just bad for you; it can quietly poison the caregiving dynamic. When you're exhausted, burned out, or running on fumes, it's easy to lash out without meaning to. That tension can cause your loved one to withdraw or avoid asking for what they need, which only makes care harder for both of you. It's a downward spiral, but it *can* be stopped. The moment you notice it, pause. Acknowledge your role, apologize if necessary, and take it as a sign that you need rest, support, and time to refill your own cup. Caring for yourself is the first step to caring for them.

Day 69

*Questions and curiosity can help manage
emotional outbursts.*

Emotional outbursts from the person you're caring for often come from a place of frustration or feeling out of control. What was once easy for them, like walking, dressing, and remembering, may now feel impossible, and that loss is painful. Instead of reacting or making assumptions about their anger or tears, approach with curiosity. Gently ask questions to help them express what's really underneath the emotion: "What's frustrating you right now?" or "How can I make this feel easier?" Questions open the door to understanding, defuse tension, and remind them that their voice and feelings still matter.

Day 70

If you run on empty for too long, you will break down.

You're not a machine, you're a miracle. But even miracles need maintenance. Skipping meals, sleep, or emotional rest may feel noble in the short term, but it's a fast track to burnout. You cannot give what you don't have. Refueling doesn't mean booking a spa weekend (though, yes please!), it means daily pauses, deep breaths, decent meals, laughter, and moments where you matter. Don't wait until you're drained to address your needs. Caregiving is a marathon, not a sprint. Build in small moments of rest now, before your body and spirit force you to. Protect your energy, it's not selfish, it's survival.

Day 71

Remember to see your doctor for yourself.

You've got appointments circled for everyone else, but what about you? Don't let your own health fall by the wayside. Caregiving is physically and emotionally taxing. You need regular checkups, screenings, and vaccines (especially flu shots) to stay strong. When you're rundown or unwell, everyone feels it. Book your physical. Keep that eye exam. Bring up that nagging issue you've been ignoring. You're not just a caregiver; you're a human who matters. The best care you can give starts with taking care of yourself. You deserve health, support, and peace of mind.

Day 72

Don't take it personally if your loved one needs a break from you.

It's not about you, it's about them. Sometimes, your loved one may need space, rest, or independence more than company. That can sting, especially when you're pouring out so much love. But try not to take it as rejection. Their request may come from fatigue, pride, confusion, or a need for control in a world where they feel powerless. Respect their wishes while reminding them you're there. Maintain a steady connection, even when you're far away. Leave a kind note. Send a small treat. Make a quick call just to say hello. Your care is still felt. You haven't failed them by stepping back. You're honoring what they need.

Day 73

Others may not understand just how difficult caregiving can be.

Others often don't realize just how demanding caregiving truly is. What seems like a simple task, like tossing in a load of laundry, can become an ordeal when clothing is stained with blood, medications, or bodily fluids and needs extra care. Even helping someone eat or get dressed can take twice as long as it might for someone healthy. When someone downplays your role with comments like, "It can't be that hard," try responding with, "Caregiving adds layers you don't see, but I'd be happy to have you join me for a day to get a real sense of it." Inviting them to lend a hand not only opens their eyes but might even earn you some much-needed support.

Day 74

Listen to your inner self... there is wisdom within.

You're surrounded by noise, opinions, to-do lists, alarms, and voices, but somewhere beneath it all, your inner self is whispering. That voice is wise. It's gathered insight from every sleepless night, every tough decision, and every quiet victory. Your intuition is more than a gut feeling; it's your soul speaking truth. Don't drown it out with doubt or comparison. Trust it. Sometimes the wisest guidance doesn't come from experts, but from within yourself. You already know more than you think. Know that the small voice in your head is your compass, and even if the path feels uncertain, it's pointing toward peace.

Day 75

You can lead someone to water, but you can't make them drink. You can, however, do things to make them thirsty.

You can't force someone to do what they're not ready or willing to do, but you can create an environment that encourages them to choose for themselves. Caregiving often means guiding with gentle influence rather than control. Instead of pushing, offer options, set up routines, and create moments that spark their willingness to engage. It's about planting seeds, making something appealing, inviting, or meaningful, so the decision feels like theirs. When you give them that sense of control, they're far more likely to lean into what's needed without resistance.

Day 76

Find your voice.

Your voice is a tool; use it. Ask the questions others avoid. Push for clarity. Say no when your plate is full. Advocating doesn't make you rude; it makes you responsible. You're the front line of support for someone who can't always speak for themselves. But don't forget to speak for yourself, too. If something feels wrong, say something. If you need help, ask. If a boundary is needed, set it. Your needs matter. Your words have weight. Don't shrink to keep things peaceful; speak up to maintain a healthy environment. Use your voice because it was made for this.

Day 77

Be kind to yourself.

Amid caregiving chaos, the person who is most often neglected is you. Your well-being isn't a luxury, it's a necessity. Kindness toward yourself starts small: a walk, a deep breath, a favorite show, a glass of something refreshing. It's giving yourself grace when things go sideways, which they inevitably will. Stay active enough to feel alive, not overwhelmed. Feed your body, your spirit, and your sense of humor. Celebrate tiny wins and moments of calm. Caregivers pour out so much; don't forget to refill your tank. Your presence is powerful, but your peace is precious. Guard both with gentleness and intention.

Day 78

Caregiving is what you do, not who you are.

Caregiving is something you *do*; it's not the whole of who you are. It's easy to let the role consume your identity, especially when every day revolves around appointments, meals, and meeting someone else's needs. But you are more than the tasks you complete or the care you give. You're still the friend, the parent, the partner, the dreamer, and the person you were before caregiving began. Holding onto that truth matters. Make space, even in small ways, to reconnect with what makes you *you*. Your identity is bigger than this chapter and keeping that perspective will help you navigate it with more balance and grace.

Day 79

Even if they forget the moment, they'll remember the feeling.

Memory may fade, but emotion lingers. A person with dementia may not remember your visit, but they'll feel your warmth long after you're gone. The music you played. The tone of your voice. The way you held their hand. These things register. They leave an imprint on their spirit, even if not on their timeline. Don't underestimate the power of presence. Just because they don't remember it doesn't mean it didn't matter. What you bring, such as your calm, your care, and your consistency, creates a kind of safety that transcends memory. Be gentle. Be kind. Your presence is still deeply felt, even when it's forgotten.

Day 80

Never be afraid to fall apart.

Falling apart feels terrifying; like losing control, failing, or unraveling beyond repair. But maybe it's also the chance to rebuild from the inside out. Not into who the world expects you to be, but into someone wiser and freer. Caregiving will test your limits and expose your raw edges. Let it. Let the pieces fall if they need to. Then gather them with intention. Rebuild with more boundaries, more softness, more joy. This isn't destruction, it's transformation. Don't fear the fall, fear staying stuck. You deserve to come back stronger, more yourself, and more beautiful.

Day 81

Put groceries on autopilot.

You don't need to spend your brainpower remembering if you have milk. Automate what you can by using online grocery apps to create recurring orders of your staples. Sign up for a weekly produce box. Keep a running list on your fridge or phone. Or better yet, delegate this one. Let someone else "own" groceries for a while. Streamlining food shopping means fewer emergency trips and less mental clutter. And when caregiving is already full of unexpected curveballs, that kind of predictability is gold. Set it, forget it, eat well, and move on to more important things.

Day 82

There is light out there, it's just blocked right now.

There is a light there, it hasn't gone out, it's just hidden behind the heavy clouds of the moment. When caregiving feels especially dark, it's easy to forget that there is still brightness to be found. But it does. Sometimes it shows up in a shared laugh, a quiet moment of connection, or a brief sigh of relief when something actually goes right. You don't have to pretend everything's fine, but you *can* look for those small glimmers. Let them remind you that even in the hard times, there's still light; even if it's sometimes faint and fleeting, it's always worth noticing.

Day 83

There is great strength in asking for help.

Help isn't a white flag; it's a power move. It takes courage to say, "I need support." And the strength to let someone into your mess. We're trained to do it all, but the truth is, caregiving is too big for one set of shoulders. Asking for help doesn't mean you're weak; it means you're wise enough to share the load. The people who love you want to help. Give them the chance and give yourself a break. Asking for help isn't failure, it's leadership. And leaders know when to call in reinforcements.

Day 84

Routines offer comfort.

Routine isn't boring, it's a lifeline. For those you're caring for, structure offers comfort. Knowing what comes next helps reduce anxiety, resistance, and confusion. For you, it provides rhythm in the chaos. Start with simple anchors: meals at consistent times, daily walks, and a set bedtime. Routine can bring calm, even when the circumstances feel unpredictable. You don't have to create a rigid schedule, just a reliable flow. In caregiving, stability is sacred. And when the world feels out of control, routine says, "Here is one thing you can count on." It doesn't have to be perfect to be powerful. Small, consistent actions make a big difference. Over time, these patterns become a source of trust, reminding both you and them that steadiness is possible, even in the most challenging of seasons.

Day 85

Never let a bad situation bring out the worst in you.

Hard days are inevitable. Tempers flare, plans fall apart, and exhaustion makes everything feel worse. But don't let the chaos around you create chaos within you. You have the power to respond with calmness, kindness, and strength, even when the situation screams otherwise. That doesn't mean you fake happiness; it means you anchor yourself in integrity. Let the challenging moments shape you, not sour you. Choose patience when it's hard, grace when it's easier to snap, and perspective when you want to spiral. Your strength isn't just in what you handle, it's in how you handle it. Stay grounded. Stay kind.

Tip: If you hit the wall and need a release, give those around you a warning. Simply say, "I'm at my wits' end and can't keep it bottled up another minute. I need to get it out, then we can move on."

Day 86

Sometimes the hardest thing and the right thing are the same.

Doing the right thing doesn't always feel noble or empowering—it can feel heartbreaking, exhausting, and lonely. Whether it's setting boundaries, having difficult conversations, or making impossible decisions, the path of integrity is often steep. But don't confuse "hard" with "wrong." In caregiving, love usually looks like sacrifice, silence, or strength you didn't know you had. Trust that the right path isn't supposed to be easy; it's meant to be true. If your actions are rooted in compassion and clarity, keep going. Even if your knees shake, even if your heart aches, right is still right.

Day 87

Swap criticism for self-love.

Caregivers are often their own harshest critics. You replay what you said, what you didn't do, or where you "should've" tried harder. Stop. That critical voice isn't helping; it's hurting. What you need is grace. You're doing the best you can under intense pressure, and that deserves tenderness, not judgment. Would you talk to a friend the way you speak to yourself? Doubt it. Offer encouragement, forgiveness, and a pat on the back, even for the small wins. Self-love isn't selfish, it's fuel. Quiet the inner critic. Turn up the volume on kindness. You are worthy of the same care you give.

Day 88

If you're in a difficult situation, step back and consider how you would advise a good friend who is having the same problem. Then take your own advice.

We are often kinder, wiser, and more reasonable with others than with ourselves. So, when you're stuck, overwhelmed, or deep in self-blame, pause. Ask: "What would I say if my best friend were in this exact spot?" Odds are, you'd offer grace, encouragement, and practical advice, not judgment or guilt. So why not provide that for yourself? Step outside your moment. See it from the eyes of someone who loves you. Then follow that counsel. You deserve the same compassion you so freely give. Be your own advocate. Be your own ally. Take your own good, loving advice.

Day 89

*The struggle you are in today is developing the
strength you need for tomorrow.*

Hardships don't feel helpful in the moment. They feel heavy,
uninvited, and often unfair. But over time, they do something
incredible—they build strength, emotional muscle, patience, and
courage. The very things you're being forced to develop right now
will carry you into future seasons with steadier hands and a softer
heart. You may not notice the growth while you're in the grind, but
one day you'll look back and realize: you became someone stronger
through it. You're not stuck; you're being shaped. The you of
tomorrow is counting on the you of today to keep showing up.

Day 90

*Mini breaks are an easy way to replenish your
energy and lower your stress.*

Don't underestimate the power of a five-minute breather. A quick
walk outside, a deep breath on the porch, a cup of tea in silence are
the small moments that restore you. You don't need a vacation to
reset; just a pause. Create mini-break rituals during the day:
stretch, journal, listen to music, close your eyes, and breathe. These
short pauses tell your body, "I see you. You matter." The stress may
not disappear, but your ability to handle it improves. Caregiving
doesn't stop, but you can step aside briefly and return stronger. Fill
your cup, even if it's only one sip at a time.

Day 91

Make sure your own legal documents are in order.

You're handling so much for someone else, but don't forget to attend to your own paperwork. Power of attorney, healthcare proxy, living will—these things matter. Life can change in an instant, and being prepared isn't pessimistic; it's empowering. Get your documents in place. Keep them updated. Let someone know where they are. It's one less thing for your family to worry about down the line. It also models responsibility toward those around you. Taking care of yourself legally is an act of love. Think of it as future you saying, "I've got this." Because you do.

Day 92

Getting into the nitty gritty helps volunteers provide better, more helpful assistance.

Don't sugarcoat your needs. When someone offers help, be specific. "Dinner would be amazing... but no onions, please." "Can you sit with Dad from 2 to 4 on Friday while I nap?" Clarity empowers action. Volunteers want to help; they just need direction. The more detailed you are, the more likely you are to get the help that helps. This isn't being bossy; it's being strategic. Think of it like giving someone a recipe instead of just saying "Make dinner." It removes guesswork, builds confidence, and creates real relief for you. Be clear, honest, and detailed. It's a gift to everyone.

Day 93

Don't sweat the small stuff.

Not every battle needs to be fought. Not every dish needs to be spotless. Some days, victory is just brushing your teeth and making it through the hour. Permit yourself to let go of the little things. When the day feels too big, zoom in. Just the next minute. Just the next breath. Courage isn't loud or perfect; it's consistent. Show up messy if you have to, but show up. Release the pressure to have it all together. You're doing a massive thing in tiny increments. Let that be enough. Keep your focus small and your heart steady.

Day 94

Focus on doing your best, and that sometimes means being real and honest about what you need.

Doing your best doesn't mean doing it all. It means showing up with honesty and heart, even when the truth is, "I can't handle this alone." Being honest about your limits is a strength, not a shortcoming. Ask for help when you're struggling. Admit when you're tired. Say, "I need a break," before you break down. You're not made of steel; you're made of love. And love honors truth. The more transparent you are about your needs, the more sustainable your care becomes. You don't have to fake fine. You have to be real... and that's more than enough.

Day 95

It doesn't get easier; you get stronger.

Let's be honest: caregiving rarely gets easier. The challenges shift, but the weight doesn't always lift. What *does* change, however, is you. You grow stronger, steadier, and more capable, even if you don't always see or feel it. What once felt overwhelming becomes something you handle with quiet confidence. That's not because the road smoothed out, it's because you did the hard work of rising to meet it. Strength doesn't shout. It shows up in the way you keep showing up. When it still feels heavy, remember you're not failing; you're getting stronger. And that strength is fast becoming your superpower.

Day 96

Grow a thick skin.

In caregiving, people will say the wrong thing. Often. Sometimes it's ignorance, sometimes it's insensitivity, or sometimes it's just someone having a worse day than you. You can't control their words or moods—but you can grow a protective layer between their noise and your peace. Thick skin doesn't mean a hard heart. It means learning to pause before reacting, to brush off the unhelpful, and to protect your own mental space. You're allowed to care deeply and still not let every comment affect you deeply. Consider it emotional SPF; it doesn't block the sun, but it prevents unnecessary burns.

Day 97

*It is ok... and, actually necessary... to take
a guilt-free break*

You don't need to "earn" rest. You don't need to feel bad for stepping away. A break isn't abandoning your role; it's reinforcing your strength. Caregiving is demanding, emotional, and all-consuming. Taking time to reset your mind and body isn't selfish, it's sustainable. Whether it's a nap, a walk, a weekend away, or just 10 minutes of silence in the car, take it. Don't spend your whole break feeling bad about needing one. The world won't crumble, and you'll come back stronger. Guilt doesn't belong in your suitcase. Pack peace, rest, and a snack instead.

Day 98

*Find someone who has traveled a similar path
but is a few steps ahead of you.*

There's nothing quite like connecting with someone who's been there, done that, and still knows where their coffee is. A person just a bit ahead of you on the caregiving journey can offer insight, encouragement, and those priceless "you're not crazy" moments. They navigated the storm, made mistakes, and discovered a few shortcuts. Their wisdom won't fix everything, but it will light your way. Let them be your lighthouse when you're feeling lost. Ask questions, borrow their tools, and lean on their hope until yours returns. They're proof that the road continues and that you're not alone on it.

Day 99

Meditation, yoga, listening to music, or simple deep breathing will help relieve stress.

You don't need a spa weekend to find relief (though, let's be honest, wouldn't that be nice?). Sometimes peace starts with a single breath. Meditation, yoga, or simply sitting quietly with your favorite playlist can help interrupt the swirl of stress, allowing your nervous system to catch its breath. Even five minutes makes a difference. These practices aren't about escaping; they're about reconnecting to yourself. Don't dismiss the simple things. Stillness is powerful. Breath is medicine. Quiet is a balm. Give yourself permission to pause, exhale, and exist without expectation. You don't have to earn your peace; it's available right now.

Day 100

Resource: aarp.org

AARP isn't just for retirement discounts. It's a caregiving powerhouse. Their website is packed with checklists, articles, and tools to help navigate elder care, long-term planning, and caregiver stress. Whether you're researching Medicare options or looking for caregiver support groups, AARP connects the dots with credibility and clarity. It's invaluable for sandwich-generation caregivers, those who care for aging parents while raising their children. The guides are practical, the tone is reassuring, and the site is refreshingly easy to navigate. It's like a digital compass pointing you toward the resources you didn't know you needed, until you needed them.

Day 101

*Miracles are all around you, but often
come in disguise.*

Not all miracles are big and flashy. Some look like a smile from someone who hasn't smiled in days. A full night's sleep. A kind word from a stranger. An unexpected laugh in the middle of hardship. When you're deep in caregiving, it's easy to miss these quiet blessings—but they're there. Watch for them. Let them soften you. Let them remind you that grace is still present. The miracle might not be a cure. It might be a moment. And those small, sacred moments have the power to sustain you through the longest days.

Day 102

Weed out negative people and friends.

When your energy is already stretched thin, the last thing you need is someone adding unnecessary drama or judgment. Not everyone deserves front-row access to your life. It's okay, essential, even, to lovingly distance yourself from people who drain your spirit. Tighten your circle. Surround yourself with encouragers, listeners, and those who uplift rather than undermine. It's not cruel, it's strategic. This season demands strength, and negativity is dead weight. You're not obligated to keep toxic people just because of history or guilt. Prune the garden of your relationships so you can grow. Healthy boundaries are love... with a backbone.

Day 103

Don't keep secrets.

You're not protecting anyone by staying silent; you're actually isolating yourself. Sharing what's happening invites support, understanding, and maybe even solutions. People can't show up if they don't know there's a need. Be honest about the tough days. Let them into the mess, not just the milestones. Vulnerability builds bridges. Secrets build walls. You don't have to tell everyone, but don't carry everything alone. Keep your circle informed. It's not drama, it's reality. And it's okay to say, "Here's what I'm going through. I could use a hand." Help is out there. But first, you've got to let people in.

Day 104

Love is one thing that cannot be taken away.

Diseases may change personalities. Memories may fade. Circumstances may unravel. But the love you pour into someone remains. Even when they can't say thank you. Even when they don't recognize your face. Your love imprints on their soul. It weaves into the spaces between the words. It is seen, felt, and carried, whether spoken or silent. Nothing can erase that. Not time. Not illness. Not distance. What you give in love, you give forever. And that is your legacy. That is your proof. That is your quiet, unstoppable power.

Day 105

When someone asks how you are doing, have a response ready that doesn't mask your struggles, but opens the door for compassion instead.

"Fine" is easy, but it's rarely true. When someone asks how you're doing, resist the reflex to gloss over your real feelings. Instead, have an honest-but-manageable answer ready: "It's been a tough week, but I'm hanging in," or "I'm stretched thin... thanks for asking." You don't owe everyone your whole story, but vulnerability invites support. Let people in, even just a little. You never know who's willing to help unless you give them the chance. Honesty doesn't make you a burden; it makes you brave. And sometimes, a simple, truthful answer can open a door to connection, compassion, or even just a well-timed hug.

Day 106

Happiness is found when you stop comparing yourself to other people.

Comparison is a thief. It doesn't just steal joy; it robs you of peace, progress, and pride in your journey. Caregiving isn't a competition, and no one else's highlight reel reflects your behind-the-scenes reality. Let it go. What you're doing—showing up, giving care, holding space—is enough. Stop measuring your worth by someone else's chapter. Your life is uniquely beautiful, messy, and full of meaning. Happiness doesn't arrive when you "catch up" to others. It arrives when you appreciate where you are, who you are, and how far you've come. Stay in your lane. Trust your pace. You're doing just fine.

Day 107

*My caregiver mantra is to remember: "The only control
you have is over the changes you choose to make."*

You can't control illness. You can't control the outcomes. But you can control your response. Your choices. Your mindset. That's your power. Focus on what you can change, such as your routines, your self-care, and your boundaries. Don't exhaust yourself trying to fix everything. Let go of the chaos you can't command and shift your energy to the areas you can influence. That's where real strength lives. Let this mantra be your anchor. Say it when things spiral: "I choose my next step." Because in the storm of caregiving, your calm, grounded choices are the most powerful thing you own.

Day 108

*Keep your eyes, ears, mind, and heart open
to offers of help.*

Help might come in unexpected ways: a neighbor dropping off soup, a coworker offering to drive, a friend checking in "just because." Stay open. Say yes. Let go of the idea that accepting help is a sign of weakness. It's wisdom. People want to show up—but they need to know it's welcome. Don't shrug off kindness or downplay your needs. Be receptive. Be grateful. Be real. Help may not solve everything, but it lightens the load. When your eyes are open to grace, it tends to show up. Help is love in motion; accept it.

Day 109

*Let go of what you cannot change and hold
on tightly to love.*

You will face things you can't fix. Declines you can't stop. Behaviors that feel unfair. Let them go. Don't waste your limited energy fighting what's beyond your control. Instead, grip tightly to the good: the laughter, the shared memories, the tiny moments of clarity or connection. That love, raw, honest, and sometimes messy, is what will carry you through the complex parts. It doesn't have to be picture-perfect to be powerful. Release the need to control everything. Embrace the love that remains. That's where the magic lives. That's what matters most.

Day 110

*Include logistical household items on your
care calendar, too.*

It's not just the "care" in caregiving; it's the life around the care that gets overwhelming. A well-thought-out care calendar helps manage the bigger picture: not just the medical needs, but also the everyday tasks that accumulate. Include meals, errands, dog walks, doctor appointments, bills, yard work, companionship visits—you name it. Break the giant list into manageable parts and assign or schedule them. Visual structure reduces mental chaos. You don't have to juggle it all. Organizing your support system keeps things from slipping through the cracks. It also makes it easier to say yes when someone asks, "How can I help?"

Day 111

Don't deny reality.

Denial may feel comforting in the short term, but it only delays the healing and preparedness that come with facing the truth. Face the situation honestly, even when it hurts. Acknowledge the hard parts and allow yourself to grieve what's changing. Then make your next move with clear eyes and a steady heart. You're not weak for naming reality. You're wise. It's from that place of truth that real strength and resilience are born. You don't have to accept every moment cheerfully, but receiving the facts gives you the power to act, plan, and love well. Reality is your anchor. Let it steady you, not sink you.

Day 112

Look ahead, but not too far ahead; it can be overwhelming.

Planning is helpful... obsessing is exhausting. In caregiving, it's tempting to try to script every future possibility mentally. But the truth? You'll burn out before you even get there. Focus on the near horizon. What needs attention today? Tomorrow? Next week at most? You can't forecast every twist and trying to will only increase your anxiety. Let the future unfold in chapters; not as one long, looming to-do list. Permit yourself to take it in smaller bites. Looking ahead is wise, but looking too far can rob you of the peace of the present. Zoom in, breathe and trust the process. One page and one day at a time.

Day 113

*Leverage TV commercials to broach
uncomfortable conversations.*

Sometimes the easiest way to start a tough conversation is to let the
TV, or even the news, do the heavy lifting. If a commercial for an
assisted living community comes on, you might casually ask,
"What do you think about a place like that?" It's a gentle way to
open the door without making it feel like an ambush. The same
goes for other sensitive topics. For example, if a news story comes
up about medical care or end-of-life planning, you could say, "I saw
that and wondered how you'd feel about something like that for
yourself." These moments create natural opportunities to talk,
without forcing the issue.

Day 114

What you give shapes your life.

Caregiving may not come with a paycheck, but it pays in deeper
currencies: love, meaning, and legacy. The things we give, such as
our time, patience, and attention, shape the kind of life we lead far
more than what we accumulate. Giving doesn't drain us when it's
done with love and balance; it fills spaces that nothing else can.
That's not to say giving is easy; sometimes it's downright
exhausting. But it's the giving that turns ordinary days into
meaningful ones. Keep perspective. You are building a life of
substance, not just survival. And in the end, what you give is what
echoes loudly and beautifully.

Day 115

Never become so consumed by trying to fix the unfixable that you forget your soul has a purpose.

Caregiving can become so consuming that it feels like your whole identity. But you are more than a fixer. You're a soul with dreams, humor, insight, and purpose beyond the caregiving role. Some things can't be changed, and trying to control them will only break your spirit. Shift your focus from fixing to being: being present, being kind, and being aware of the deeper meaning in the moment. You're not just helping someone live; you're still living, too. And your soul needs room to breathe. Don't lose yourself in what can't be changed. Find yourself in what still matters.

Day 116

Create a caregiving team comprised of truly caring, nurturing individuals.

You don't need a crowd; you need a crew. Build a team around you with people who genuinely care, not just those who feel obligated. Look for calm voices, steady hands, flexible minds, and kind hearts. They don't all need medical degrees, just reliability, empathy, and the willingness to show up. Some may cook. Others may clean. Someone may sit beside you and make you laugh. You deserve support from people who bring peace, not pressure. Let go of toxic help. Invite in the nurturing kind. Caregiving isn't meant to be a solo act; it's a community of compassion in motion.

Day 117

Delegate tasks to others who are capable.

You don't have to do it all. Really. Even if you're the MVP of multitasking, trying to carry every responsibility yourself is a straight shot to burnout. Look around—some people want to help, but don't know how. Let them. Whether it's asking a neighbor to pick up groceries or letting a sibling handle an appointment, delegation isn't weakness; it's wisdom. Trust others with part of the load. The world won't crumble. Sure, they may not accomplish the task the exact way you would have, but if it's done, it's done. You deserve a bit of time in your day and space in your mind. Don't wear "I do everything" like a badge of honor. Let others show up and share the load.

Day 118

Learn how to cope productively and successfully with crisis.

Crisis has a way of showing up uninvited and overstaying its welcome. You can't always prevent chaos, but you can train yourself to respond with resilience instead of panic. Coping productively means finding what works for you: breathing exercises, journaling, prayer, music, or movement. It's about creating a personal emergency kit, not of bandages, but of habits that keep you grounded. Coping doesn't mean pretending everything's fine; it means acknowledging reality and choosing to face it with tools, not just tears. Build your inner toolbox. When crisis hits (and it will), you'll be ready; maybe not perfect, but you will be prepared, and that's powerful.

Day 119

It can be comforting and refreshing to speak with others who share your caregiving experience.

There's nothing like being around people who truly understand. You don't have to explain the fatigue or the quiet grief behind the smile. Whether it's a virtual group, a conference breakout session, or chatting over coffee with someone who's been there, a shared experience is soul fuel. It reminds you that you're not isolated or invisible. You're part of a compassionate community. So, make time for connection. Those conversations can be more healing than any medicine. Sometimes the best therapy is someone who nods and says, "Me too."

Day 120

Find the funny in everything.

Humor doesn't cancel the hard stuff; it helps carry it. In caregiving, absurdity shows up daily. Milk is in the pantry. Shoes are in the fridge. A heartfelt conversation with a talking pill bottle. Instead of losing your mind, try laughing, not at the person, but at the situation. Finding humor doesn't mean you're not taking things seriously; it means you're permitting yourself to breathe. Comedy is the pressure valve that keeps the soul from exploding. Look for the ridiculous. Smile at the chaos. If you can't find the funny, be the funny. You'll survive longer and with better stories to tell later.

Day 121

Read: Helping Yourself Help Others by Rosalynn Carter

Former First Lady Rosalynn Carter was not just a public servant—she was a caregiver herself. Her book is a powerful blend of research, personal insight, and advocacy. It reminds you that caregiving is a societal issue, not just a personal one. If you feel like the system isn't designed with you in mind, you're right; and Carter gives language and encouragement for that truth. She speaks to both your heart and your brain, helping you take care of yourself while you care for someone else. It's both a balm and a blueprint.

Day 122

Don't argue! Do what's best for the one who needs the care.

You won't always agree—and that's okay. But caregiving isn't about winning debates. It's about choosing what brings the most dignity, peace, and safety to the person in your care. When emotions run high, pause. Breathe. Ask, "Is this about being right... or being kind?" Arguments drain energy you could use for more meaningful moments. Sometimes, doing what's best doesn't look like what everyone wants, but it's rooted in love. Let compassion lead, not ego. Peace over power. Care over control. You're not just helping them—you're protecting the heart of the relationship. And that matters more than being "right."

Day 123

Be there for others but never leave yourself behind.

You're generous with your care, but don't abandon yourself in the process. Show up for others, yes—but keep showing up for yourself too. It's not selfish to protect your needs. Pouring from an empty cup helps no one. Pause, breathe, and ask, "What do I need today?" Even if the answer is five minutes of silence or a sandwich you didn't have to share. You deserve the same compassion you give so freely. Be present for others but anchor yourself first. You can be kind and still have boundaries. You can be giving and still be whole. Stay in your own corner.

Day 124

One small positive thought in the morning can change your entire day.

Before your feet hit the floor, give your mind a moment of kindness. One small, intentional thought, such as "I can handle what comes," or "Today is a fresh start," can rewire your outlook. It doesn't need to be a formal speech, just a gentle nudge toward hope. That single thought can act like emotional coffee, waking up the part of you that still believes in good things. Will it erase all stress? No. But it shifts your posture toward the day. You get to decide the first message your brain receives. Make it something that lifts, steadies, or encourages you. Tiny thought... big impact.

Day 125

There will be people who avoid the topic and your situation; that's OK... but you might need to limit your interaction with them.

Some people disappear when things get hard. They don't know what to say, or your reality makes them uncomfortable. That doesn't mean you've done anything wrong. Not everyone is equipped to walk beside you. And that's okay. You don't need a crowd; you need a circle. A few trusted people who show up, ask the right questions, or simply stay. If someone's absence stings, grieve it, but don't chase them. Instead, invest your energy where love is present, where understanding flows, and where you're not just tolerated, but seen. That's the company your heart deserves.

Day 126

Collaborative caregiving ensures all voices are heard.

Collaborative caregiving means involving your loved one in decisions about their care whenever possible. Let them share their preferences, fears, and opinions; it gives them a sense of control and dignity during a time when so much feels out of their hands. But collaboration doesn't mean agreeing to everything; ultimately, you're responsible for making choices that are right and safe. The key is *how* you approach it. When you act like a dictator, it only breeds resistance and resentment. When you invite their input, listen with respect, and explain your reasoning, you build trust and create a care plan that feels supportive rather than imposed.

Day 127

Resource: www.caregiveraction.org

This resource is built by caregivers for caregivers. The Caregiver Action Network offers emotional support, practical advice, and valuable resources without sugarcoating the challenging aspects. They recognize caregiving as real work, and they treat it with the dignity it deserves. You'll find webinars, checklists, peer stories, and access to a free Caregiver Help Desk for personalized help. It's especially useful if you're caring for someone with a serious illness or chronic condition. Their motto is "You are not alone," and they back it up with real-time support and practical wisdom.

Day 128

Take one day at a time.

When life gets overwhelming, take a step back. Don't try to solve next month's challenges with today's energy. Just focus on this hour. This breath. This is the next right step. You don't have to have a five-year plan—you need to make it to lunch. The beauty of one-day-at-a-time living is that it keeps you present, grounded, and sane. Some days, getting out of bed is the win. Other days, it's managing a complete to-do list... both count. You don't have to sprint through life. You can walk gently, moment by moment. Focus on managing this day; tomorrow can wait its turn.

Day 129

Make friends with good-hearted people.

Your tribe matters. In caregiving, your emotional environment can either lift you or sink you. Surround yourself with kind souls; the ones who check in, show up, and offer love without an agenda. These people are emotional oxygen. Good-hearted friends don't need perfect explanations; they just get it. They won't judge your exhaustion or your messy house. They'll bring snacks, shoulders, and sometimes sarcasm. Friendship isn't about frequency; it's about authenticity. Find the ones who remind you of who you are beneath the stress. Let them in. You're not meant to carry this alone. Good hearts recognize other good hearts.

Day 130

Cut yourself some slack!

Perfection is a trap—and you don't have time for it. Let go of the idea that everything must be spotless, perfectly planned, and picture-perfect. Some days, success looks like cereal for dinner and everyone staying safe. That's okay. Lower the bar. Then sit on it, have a snack, and exhale. You're doing enough... actually, more than enough. Don't measure your worth by your productivity. Measure it by your presence, your heart, or your resilience. Be kind to yourself. You'd forgive a friend for missing a beat, so do the same for yourself. And remember, grace over guilt... always.

Day 131

*Giving doesn't empty you; it grows you, as long
as you protect it with healthy boundaries.*

Giving time, attention, or love doesn't deplete us the way we fear it will. In fact, giving expands us. It makes our hearts softer and our souls stronger. But here's the key: healthy giving comes with boundaries. You can be generous and still say no. You can care deeply and still protect your peace. The wealthiest people aren't those with full calendars, they're those with full hearts. You're giving in ways few people understand, and it matters. You're not losing anything by loving this hard. You're becoming someone stronger and kinder. That's a type of wealth that never runs out.

Day 132

Don't harbor resentment. Start each day fresh.

Resentment can quietly poison your days if you let it take root. It's natural to feel hurt, disappointed, or frustrated. Those emotions are part of being human. But holding on to them only keeps you stuck in the past, draining the energy you need for today. Letting go isn't about pretending it didn't happen; it's about choosing not to let it control you. Each day presents an opportunity to release what no longer serves you and step forward with a clearer, lighter heart. Ask yourself what you need to reset and focus on what truly matters now.

Day 133

Compassion heals what judgment never can.

Judgment creates divides, while compassion builds bridges. When someone is struggling, especially someone in your care, they don't need correction. They need connection. A soft word, a gentle tone, or a moment of understanding does more to heal than a thousand lectures. That includes how you speak to yourself, too. Condemning yourself for what you missed or messed up only deepens the wound. But compassion? It invites healing. It says, "You're still worthy." Caregiving isn't about getting it all right; it's about loving well, even when it's hard. Choose the path that opens hearts, rather than hardening them.

Day 134

Accepting help doesn't make you weak,
it shows how strong you are.

Asking for help can feel like surrendering, but it's one of the bravest things you can do. You don't lose strength by leaning on others; you gain support. It takes courage to admit you're tired, overextended, or in need of backup. Accepting help isn't defeat; it's strategic delegation with a side of self-preservation. Let someone cook, clean, or sit beside you. It doesn't make you less capable, it proves you're wise enough to know your limits. Strong people know when to carry and when to share the weight. Let go of the guilt. Open your hands and let them help.

Day 135

Develop good time management skills.

Time doesn't bend for anyone, but how you manage it can make or break your day. Caregiving demands juggling meds, appointments, meals, and emotions. Without a plan, you'll feel like you're always playing catch-up. Try lists, calendars, alarms, or even color-coded sticky notes if that works for you. Protect your time like you would someone else's because you deserve efficiency and breathing room. Learn to say no when needed. Schedule rest like it's a priority (because it is). Good time management isn't about doing more; it's about doing what matters most. With one well-planned day at a time, you can take back control and find a little calm.

Day 136

Admit you do not know all the answers.

No one has all the answers, especially in the messy world of caregiving. You're not failing. You just don't know everything; you're learning. Asking questions, making mistakes, and adapting on the fly is wisdom in motion. Permit yourself not to know. To say, "I don't have that figured out yet." No shame. No guilt. Let it be a doorway, not a dead end. The most compassionate people are often the most curious. So, stay humble. Stay teachable. You'll gain more peace from honesty than you ever will from pretending to have it all together. You don't; and that's okay.

Day 137

Sometimes the best thing you can do is keep going.

When you're bone-tired, maxed out, and feeling like you're out of moves, consider this: forward is forward, even if you're crawling. Bravery isn't always loud or flashy. Sometimes it's dragging yourself out of bed, answering one email, or sitting in silence so you don't snap. That *is* strength. Don't wait for perfect conditions or a lightning bolt of clarity. Take the next step, however small or shaky. It might not look like much, but it counts. Every step builds momentum, and every choice stacks up. You don't need a five-year plan right now; you just need the guts to take the next move.

Day 138

Check into services such as transportation, meal delivery, and housekeeping to lighten the load.

You don't have to do it all. There are local and national services that can lighten your load; transportation programs, meal delivery, respite care, and housekeeping help. These services aren't handouts; they're lifelines. Ask your doctor, social worker, or local aging center for recommendations. Use websites like Eldercare.gov or your insurance portal to search for support. Help isn't a luxury; it's part of sustainable caregiving. Let others step in where they can, so you can step back when needed. Take advantage of what's out there. It doesn't mean you care less; it means you care wisely. You are allowed to be supported.

Day 139

Appreciate and schedule rest.

Rest isn't a reward you earn after a job well done; it's a necessity you schedule to survive the job itself. Caregivers often push through fatigue as if it were a badge of honor. But burnout doesn't ask permission. Rest before you hit the wall. Schedule it like any other priority. A nap, a walk, a quiet cup of tea or whatever resets your spirit. Rest is where your strength regenerates, your mind clears, and your heart softens again. It's not laziness, it's maintenance. You wouldn't run a car without gas. Don't run your life without rest. You're allowed to pause. More than allowed; you need to.

Day 140

Be stubborn about your goals and flexible about your methods.

Your goal might be clear—peace, balance, healing—but how do you get there? That's where the real magic (and messiness) happens. Life rarely sticks to Plan A, especially in caregiving. Be fierce about where you're headed, but gentle with how you get there. Adjust the route or take the detour. Maybe try a new tool. Flexibility isn't failure, it's wisdom. Being stubborn with your methods will burn you out. Being creative with your approach is key to surviving and succeeding. Don't let pride block progress. When your goal stays steady, the path is totally up for adjustment. Even when you adapt and pivot, you're still moving forward.

Day 141

You can't do it all at once, but you can do what matters most in the moment.

If you're part of the sandwich generation caring for your children while also supporting aging parents, you're juggling two full-time roles that rarely sync up. One moment you're helping with homework, the next you're navigating Medicare or managing medications. It's exhausting, emotionally complex, and often thankless. But here's the truth: you don't have to do it all at once. You can do what matters most in each moment. Some days, your kids will need your full focus. Other days, it's your parents who need extra care. That constant shifting isn't a sign of failure, it's a mark of resilience, and love that stretches across generations.

Day 142

Create a list of things you could use help with and print or write the list on business cards.

When someone says, "Let me know how I can help," your brain probably goes blank from decision fatigue. Skip the brain fog and get practical. Write down specific, helpful tasks (such as walking the dog, mowing the lawn, or sitting with Mom for an hour) and print or write them on cards. When someone offers help, hand them a card. Boom! No fumbling, no stress, no guesswork. This makes it easier for others to step up and helps you avoid the awkward "I don't know" moment. People do want to help. Give them the opportunity in a way that helps you. Smart, clear, and oh-so-liberating.

Day 143

Be the reason that someone smiles today.

Kindness doesn't need an occasion; it just needs intention. Hold a door. Offer a compliment. Leave a funny sticky note or text a GIF that makes someone laugh out loud. Caregiving can feel heavy, but small acts of joy are light enough to carry; and powerful enough to lift. Be the reason someone's hard day feels less hard. It won't fix the world, but it will ripple goodness into it. You never know who needed that moment of warmth, that smile, that reminder they're seen. Offering that smile doesn't cost anything, but it makes an impact every time.

Day 144

You can be both a good parent and a good caregiver at the same time.

Being a parent is already a full-time, heart-full role. Add caregiving to the mix, and it can feel like you're constantly falling short in one area or the other. But here's the truth; you can be both. Your love doesn't divide between roles; it multiplies. Some days, your attention will lean more toward one than the other, and that's okay. Being present, even in imperfect ways, still matters deeply. You're modeling empathy, resilience, and dedication for your children while also honoring the needs of your loved one. Don't let guilt tell you you're failing. You're showing up, twice over, with a heart that's doing its absolute best.

Day 145

No matter how tall the mountain, it cannot block the sun. — Chinese proverb

---

Challenges in caregiving can feel like a mountain: diagnoses, tough decisions, or sheer exhaustion that towers over everything. They can make you feel small and overwhelmed, but the key is to take them one step at a time. You don't have to conquer the whole mountain today; just focus on the next step forward. Rest when you need to, regroup when it's hard, but don't stop moving. Even in the hardest seasons, there are small moments of light; kindness, relief, or a quiet win that remind you why you keep going. The climb is hard, but every bit of progress matters.

Day 146

Emotions will rise and fall—find your steady rock and stand firm.

Caregiving is a wild emotional ride — one minute you're feeling grateful, the next you're Googling "how to cry quietly in a bathroom stall." The highs and lows aren't proof you're doing it wrong; they're just part of the deal. What keeps you steady is having a rock — some person, habit, or little ritual that pulls you back when the waves hit. Maybe it's your best friend. Maybe it's a quiet walk. Maybe it's your faith or just scribbling it all out in a journal. Whatever helps you stay grounded when everything else feels like quicksand — hold onto it. You don't have to be perfect or unshakable. You just need something or someone you can lean on.

Day 147

Whatever you're facing today, keep going.
Keep moving. Keep hoping.

Some days will feel heavy, as if every task requires twice the effort. On those days, focus on just one small, doable step: making a healthy meal, finishing one chore, or taking a five-minute break to breathe. On other days, you may feel lighter, giving you the energy to do a little more. Both days matter. Progress in caregiving isn't about perfection; it's built in small, consistent moments of showing up. Celebrate the little wins: a calm conversation, a smile from your loved one, or simply getting through a tough day. Those are victories, even if they don't feel big. Keep moving forward, step by step, because every effort you make is shaping a better tomorrow.

Day 148

Don't compare yourself to others.

Comparison is a one-way ticket to burnout. It's tempting to look at other caregivers and think, "They're doing better." But you're only seeing a snapshot—not the whole, unfiltered story. Your path is yours alone. It's shaped by your unique approach, your pace, and your strengths. Don't measure your progress by someone else's mile markers. Instead, reflect on where you've been and how far you've come. Celebrate your wins, no matter how small. You don't need to be anyone else; you need to keep showing up as yourself. Comparison steals joy. Compassion, especially toward yourself, brings it back.

Day 149

*When you feel small and insignificant, remember
the mighty oak was once a tiny nut.*

You may feel that your work is invisible, insignificant, mundane, and unappreciated. But small acts stack up. A hand held. A meal made. A gentle word in a hard moment. These are seeds. They don't bloom overnight, but they grow deep roots. The most significant impact often begins in the quietest places. Keep doing the small things with great love. That's where real transformation begins. Remember, the mighty oak didn't shoot up in a day. It started as something small, overlooked... even a little nutty. Sound familiar? Your care matters; even when no one's clapping. Keep planting your seeds, because the forest is forming.

Day 150

*Watch out for signs of depression and don't wait
to get professional help.*

Sadness is part of caregiving. But if it lingers, numbs, or isolates you, it might be more than just a rough patch. Watch for signs: loss of interest in things you once loved, changes in sleep or appetite, or the feeling that you're just going through the motions. This isn't a weakness, it's a signal. And the brave thing is reaching out. Counselors, therapists, and support groups aren't luxuries; they're lifelines. You don't need to hit rock bottom to ask for help. Be proactive. You matter too much to fade into the background of your own life. Help is available if you reach out for it.

Day 151

Find someone who can give you a break regularly.

You need a break—no justification required. Having someone reliable to step in, even for an hour, can breathe life back into your soul. Seek them out. Train them if needed. Trade favors. Pay if you must. But do not wear yourself out trying to do it all alone. You don't need a parade, you just need someone who knows the routine, respects your time, and says, "Go. I've got this." Consistent breaks prevent burnout. They're not selfish. They're strategic. Your sanity, sleep, and sense of humor depend on it. You can't pour from an empty pitcher.

Day 152

Check the Administration on Aging (AAA) for resources like respite care (to give yourself a break), meal plans, mobility assistance, housing and caregiver training.

You don't have to figure this all out alone. The Administration on Aging (through your local Area Agency on Aging) offers real help: respite care to give you a break, meal programs, transportation, housing support, and even training to make your caregiving safer and smoother. These services exist for you. Many are free or low-cost—so ask, explore, and apply. You've already got enough on your plate. Don't let pride or paperwork stop you from accessing what you're entitled to. Support is out there. You just have to raise your hand and say, "Yes, please."

Day 153

*If you start feeling overwhelmed or angry,
find a release or a counselor.*

Anger and overwhelm aren't character flaws—they're warning lights. When you find yourself snapping over toast or tearing up in the cereal aisle, it's time to pause. These emotions are valid, but they need somewhere safe to land. Don't bottle them. Talk to a trusted friend. Journal. Walk. Scream into a pillow. And if that's not enough, get professional help. Counselors aren't for "broken" people; they're for smart people who know they can't carry everything alone. Let someone help you sort out the mess. You're not weak, you're human. Feel the feelings, then release them and keep going with a clearer heart.

Day 154

*I hope you're proud of yourself for the times you said Yes
when it meant extra work but was helpful to someone else.*

You didn't have to say yes, but you did. And not because it was easy. You said yes when you were tired, overwhelmed, or already carrying too much. Why? Because someone needed you. That kind of heart is rare. Be proud of that. Yes, it added more to your plate, but it also added more to someone else's peace. You made their burden lighter, even for a moment. Don't downplay it. These quiet sacrifices may go unnoticed by others, but they echo in the lives you touch. You gave of yourself, and that is something to celebrate. Quiet heroes like you change everything.

Day 155

The Bible can be comforting. If you are not used to the formal language, The Message is written in layman's language.

Whether you grew up steeped in scripture or feel unsure around it, the Bible can offer deep comfort during caregiving. The Message version puts timeless truths in everyday language with no decoding required. Psalms become personal prayers, Proverbs become lifelines, and Jesus' compassion becomes deeply relevant. Even if you're not religious, these pages hold ancient wisdom about patience, suffering, and love that transcends belief. Open it when you feel lost, angry, or in need of hope. It's not about memorizing verses, it's about finding yourself in the middle of them.

Day 156

Whatever you're going through, know that many others have experienced the same and got out of it just fine.

It's easy to feel like you're the only one walking through this kind of storm. But you're not. Others have been where you are—overwhelmed, uncertain, completely spent—and they made it through. That doesn't make your pain less valid, but it reminds you that survival (and even joy) is possible. People do get through this. Not because it's easy, but because they keep choosing one more breath, one more step, one more day. Look for their stories, let their strength remind you of your own, take comfort in knowing that "through" is a real direction and you are headed there.

Day 157

"Compassion is the radicalism of our time."
— Dalai Lama

In a world that often prioritizes speed, achievement, and appearance, choosing compassion is a revolutionary act. It says, "I see you," when others look away. It slows down in a culture of rush. In caregiving, compassion is your rebellion against burnout, frustration, and isolation. It brings humanity back into the challenging moments. You're not weak for leading with heart, you're brave. You're not naive, you're intentional. When you choose compassion, even when it's hard, you're doing something radical. Let your caregiving be a quiet protest against apathy. That's the kind of revolution the world desperately needs.

Day 158

No act of kindness, no matter how small, is ever wasted.

You might think that tiny gesture didn't matter, such a kind word, a warm blanket or a shared laugh, but it did. Kindness has a ripple effect you may never fully see. It softens moments, shifts moods, and leaves a mark deeper than you know. Every small act says, "You matter." And when you give it freely, it says, "I matter, too." Even on your hardest days, kindness keeps you tethered to what's real. Whether or not it's returned or noticed, kindness always lands somewhere meaningful. It's never wasted. It may be the most powerful thing you do all day.

Day 159

Not every problem can be solved easily. Get creative!

Not every problem in caregiving has an easy fix, but creativity can open doors where frustration closes them. If your loved one resists bathing, try turning it into a soothing "spa" experience with soft music and warm towels. If taking medication is a struggle, consider pairing it with a favorite snack or using a pillbox with bright colors as a visual cue. When communication is hard, photos, music, or simple hand squeezes can speak louder than words. Creativity isn't about having all the answers; it's about staying flexible and trying new angles until something works. Small adjustments can transform overwhelming moments into ones that feel lighter and more manageable.

Day 160

Don't be afraid to say what you want, it's the only way you'll get it.

Waiting for someone to guess what you need? That's a recipe for frustration. Whether it's a break, an extra hand, or a simple hug, say it out loud. Even the most caring people can't read your mind. Asking for what you need isn't selfish, it's honest and healthy. Start small if it feels uncomfortable; even saying it out loud to yourself can build confidence. Your needs matter just as much as anyone else's and voicing them doesn't make you demanding; it makes you clear. Your voice is valuable, and it deserves to be heard.

Day 161

Caring is helping... no matter how tired you are.

Caring doesn't stop just because you're exhausted—and that's what makes it both beautiful and challenging. Even on the days when you're running on fumes, your presence, your effort, and your love still make a difference. Sometimes caring looks like big, selfless acts; other times it's simply showing up, offering a kind word, or holding a hand. Remember, it's not about doing it all perfectly; it's about giving what you can, even when you're tired. When you've done that, permit yourself to rest. Refueling is part of caring, too.

Day 162

Learn a few calming breathing techniques to soothe the mind and body.

When everything feels overwhelming and your nerves are frayed, your breath is your built-in reset button. Learning just a few calming breathing techniques can help quiet the mind, relax your body, and bring you back to center, with no equipment required. Whether it's box breathing, a slow inhale through the nose and long exhale through the mouth, or simply counting to four with each breath, these small practices can make a big difference. In the middle of chaos, your breath can be your calm. Give yourself permission to pause and breathe deeply, intentionally, often. You deserve that moment of peace.

Box breathing: 1) Inhale through your nose for four seconds; 2) hold your breath for four seconds; 3) exhale slowly through your mouth for four seconds; 4) hold again with empty lungs for four seconds.

Day 163

Each storm teaches you how to navigate.

Caregiving rarely offers calm waters. It's filled with sudden storms like emotional upheavals, physical exhaustion, and practical challenges you never saw coming. But every rough patch is teaching you something: how to adapt, how to steady yourself, and how to keep moving even when the waves feel relentless. These moments, as hard as they are, build resilience and sharpen your instincts in ways calm days never could. You're learning to navigate with strength and grace, even when the path is unclear. The next time a storm rolls in, remember, you've weathered others before, and you have the skills and grit to handle this one too.

Day 164

It may be hard to imagine leaving your loved one in someone else's care, but taking a break can be one of the best things you do for both of you.

No one else will do it exactly like you. But that doesn't mean they can't do it well enough. Letting someone else step in gives you the chance to recharge and gives your loved one someone with a new face, fresh energy, maybe even a different kind of connection. You are not abandoning them. You're investing in your ability to keep showing up. Breaks make better caregivers. And your loved one may benefit from seeing that care can come from many places, not just one superhero in disguise. Trust the process. Breathe. You both need this.

Day 165

When in doubt, take the next small step.

When you're unsure what to do, focus on the smallest step you can take. Caregiving can feel like a maze of decisions, and waiting for the "perfect" plan often leads to feeling stuck. Instead, ask yourself, "What's one thing I can do right now to make this moment better?" It might be as simple as making a list, sending a text for support, or taking a five-minute break to regroup. Small steps create clarity and momentum. You don't need to have all the answers; you just need to keep moving forward, one thoughtful step at a time. Each choice, however small, is progress, and progress builds confidence. Over time, those tiny steps stitch together into real change, showing you that forward is always possible.

Day 166

People love human touch: a handshake,
a hug, or a pat on the back.

Never underestimate the power of a simple touch. A gentle hand on a shoulder, a quick hug, or a reassuring pat can say, "I see you," in a way that words can't. In caregiving, touch becomes both practical and deeply personal because it can comfort and connect. And it goes both ways: the person you're caring for needs it, but so do you. Don't shy away from these tiny gestures. They're reminders of our shared humanity. When words fail, or emotions run high, touch steps in. It grounds, heals, and opens hearts. In those quiet moments, touch becomes a language of love that lingers long after the moment has passed.

Day 167

The first people to help you up are the ones who know what it feels like to fall down.

Genuine empathy doesn't come from pity; it comes from experience. The ones who show up when you're at your lowest are often the ones who've been there themselves. They don't flinch at your mess because they remember their own. Let them help. Let them sit beside your struggle without needing to fix it. These are the people who understand without explanation. And one day, you'll return the favor by lifting someone else with the wisdom and tenderness you earned the hard way. Or, by sending them a copy of this book. Fall if you must, but don't stay down. Hands are reaching for you, and some of them truly understand.

Day 168

The only constant 'Normal' is the setting on the washing machine.

In caregiving, "normal" is constantly shifting. Just when you think you've found a routine or a rhythm, something changes; a new medication, a sudden health issue, or an emotional curveball. It can be frustrating to realize there's no true "normal" to hold onto, but that's where flexibility becomes your greatest strength. The only real constant is your ability to adapt, even when it's uncomfortable. So instead of chasing a fixed idea of normal, focus on what works *today*. Tomorrow might look different, but that's okay, you'll adjust, just as you always have.

Day 169

If you can't find your way out of difficulty, you're probably looking for the easy way.

When you're stuck in the middle of a difficult situation, it's tempting to believe there's an easy way out, but caregiving rarely works like that. The truth is that the "easy way" often doesn't exist. Challenges in this journey require patience, persistence, and a willingness to take the hard, sometimes uncomfortable steps. Instead of searching for a shortcut, focus on the next right action, even if it's tough. The path through difficulty often looks like small, steady efforts, and while it might not feel easy, it will get you where you need to go. Each hard choice you make becomes proof of your strength and commitment. Over time, those steady efforts build not only solutions, but also resilience you may not have realized you had.

Day 170

Read a chapter of a favorite book.

Books are time machines, escape hatches, and brain vacations. Whether it's a deep, meaningful memoir or a ridiculous rom-com full of clichés, let yourself get lost in a story. Reading gives your mind a break from reality while feeding your imagination and restoring your spirit. Just one chapter can create a pocket of peace in a chaotic day. Don't feel guilty for escaping; it's nourishment. Choose something that makes you laugh, cry, or forget the laundry for a while. The world will still be there when you return, but you will be more centered when you do.

Day 171

Continue expanding your personal and professional networks.

Your world shouldn't shrink just because your responsibilities have grown. Caregiving can feel isolating, but staying connected both personally and professionally is vital. Friendships offer comfort. Professional circles offer opportunities. Both offer perspective. Make time to meet new people, even virtually. Ask questions. Swap stories. Share tips. Building your network doesn't mean being social 24/7; it means maintaining lifelines for support, learning, and perhaps even laughter. Every new connection is a thread that weaves into a safety net. You never know which relationship will bring the insight, job lead, or moment of comic relief you need. Keep the doors open.

Day 172

Tough times never last.

Storms pass, even the wildest ones. And the reason they pass isn't always because things change, it's because you grow stronger in the middle of them. Tough times test your patience, your heart, and your limits. But they also build resilience, empathy, and a kind of quiet courage that no easy day ever could. You don't have to like the hard days, but trust that they're shaping something powerful in you. You're tougher than you think. Not because you feel strong every moment, but because you keep going. That's the grit that outlasts the storm. You won't just survive, you'll rise.

Day 173

Caregiver resource: Make-A-Wish Foundation

If you're caring for a child with a critical illness, the Make-A-Wish Foundation can bring joy in ways you never imagined. Wishes aren't just a nice distraction; they're powerful moments that provide hope, strength, and emotional healing. It's a reminder that even in the middle of medical schedules and uncertainty, there's still space for magic. Reach out, learn what qualifies, and apply. You're not taking anything away from someone else; you're creating a memory your loved one will cherish forever. You don't have to do it alone. Let this beautiful organization help create something extraordinary in your journey.

Day 174

Be honest with yourself and acknowledge what you know and don't know.

You don't have to pretend to know everything. You're not a walking medical encyclopedia, emotional guru, or superhero. You're a human navigating complexity, and honesty is your best tool. Be honest with yourself. What do you know? What do you still need help with? Naming the gaps doesn't weaken you; it empowers you to grow, ask for support, and protect your energy. Self-awareness is strength in action. Be humble, not helpless. Say, "I don't know, but I'll find out," and feel your confidence expand. Clarity is kind to both yourself and to others. Keep learning. Keep asking.

Day 175

*Sometimes you have to laugh instead of cry...
or cry yourself into a laughing fit. Both are OK.*

Emotions are a wild ride, and caregiving gives you the VIP pass. One minute you're sobbing into a dish towel, the next you're cracking up over something completely absurd. Let it happen. Laughter isn't denial, it's survival. And crying? That's just emotional housekeeping. Both are valid, and they sometimes appear in the same breath. Don't overthink it. Permit yourself to feel all the feelings. Whether you're laughing, crying, or doing a bit of both at once, you're simply processing the weight of it all. It's not weird, it's healing. Let the tears fall. Let the laughter rise. You're doing great.

Day 176

Get outside or open the windows every day.

Nature has a way of putting things into perspective that is truly magical. Open a window, take a short walk, or step outside and breathe in something that isn't recycled stress. Fresh air can't solve every problem, but it can remind your body it's alive and worthy of rest. Let the wind clear your mind. Let the sunlight warm your worries. Even a few minutes outside can shift your mood and bring your thoughts back to center. You don't need an elaborate plan, just a willingness to step out and let the world do a little healing on your behalf.

Day 177

*When life changes to be harder, change
yourself to be stronger.*

When life gets harder, it's not about wishing things back to how they were; it's about finding the strength to rise to the new reality. Caregiving asks you to grow in ways you never expected—mentally, emotionally, and even physically. Strength doesn't show up all at once; it's built in the quiet moments when you keep going, even when it feels impossible. You adapt, you learn, and you discover a resilience you didn't know you had. You can't always control the challenges, but you *can* control how you respond, and each small act of courage makes you stronger.

Day 178

*There will come a time when your loved one will
be gone, and you will find comfort in the fact
that you were their caregiver.*

Someday, when the dishes are clean and the house is quiet, you'll look back—not at the chaos, but at the care. You'll remember your presence more than your perfection. You'll know you did your best, even when it was messy, hard, or thankless. You'll feel a deep, quiet peace because you showed up. Not everyone can say that. Your love was a daily action, a thousand small moments stitched together into something eternal. And long after they're gone, that love will remain with you, in you, and because of you. In the end, it won't be the chores or the challenges you remember most, but the bond you built in the midst of them.

Day 179

We are all faced with a series of great opportunities brilliantly disguised as impossible situations.

Life has a sneaky way of wrapping breakthroughs in chaos. That situation you're staring down, the one that looks impossible, overwhelming, or downright unfair, may hold something valuable. Not because it's easy, but because it forces you to dig deeper, stretch farther, and trust more. Every challenge you've faced has shaped you in ways you couldn't see at the time. Don't rush past the discomfort. Look closer. There might be a lesson, a strength, or a new version of yourself waiting on the other side. Opportunities often show up dressed like disasters. And still, you're ready for it. Even now.

Day 180

Set aside time each week for connecting, even if it's just a walk with a friend.

Isolation is sneaky. It shows up slowly, disguised as busyness and fatigue, until one day you realize you've been running on empty with no one to talk to. Don't wait for a crisis to reach out. Make connecting with others a ritual. A walk, a call, even a five-minute text exchange can remind you that you exist beyond your caregiving role. Connection recharges you. It reminds you you're human, lovable, and not alone. You don't need a big social calendar, just need a little regular warmth. You deserve to feel seen. Schedule the soul hug.

Day 181

Done is better than perfect.

"Done is better than perfect" isn't a cop-out, it's a lifeline for caregivers. When you're juggling medications, appointments, meals, and emotions, chasing perfection will only leave you drained and defeated. The truth is, your loved one doesn't need flawless; they need you present, steady, and real. A meal reheated in the microwave is still a meal. A home that's lived-in is still full of love. What matters most is that you're showing up. Release the impossible standard and honor the effort you bring each day. Trust that "good enough," done with care, is more than enough. Perfection is a myth; presence is the gift. And in the long run, it's the love behind your actions that will be remembered, not whether they were flawless.

Day 182

Believe in yourself.

You've made it through 100% of your hardest days. That's not chance, it's proof of your strength. You may not feel unstoppable every day, but that doesn't make your courage any less real. You're learning, growing, and showing up in ways most people will never witness. That's not small, it's extraordinary. Doubt may knock on the door, but don't invite it to stay. Trade fear for faith, even if your faith trembles. You've got this; not perfectly, not easily, but honestly and with heart. Trust the version of you that keeps moving forward, even when it's hard. That version is alive, steady, and braver than you give yourself credit for. And each day you rise again, you're building a strength that no setback can erase.

Day 183

Find time to be alone every day.

Solitude is not selfish, it's sacred. In the noise of caregiving, where others' needs constantly take center stage, you must carve out space just for yourself. Even ten minutes of quiet can act like a mental reset button. Use that time to breathe, think, cry, nap, pray, doodle; do whatever feeds your soul. It's not about isolation; it's about restoration. This isn't extra credit, it's essential maintenance. You don't need to disappear for hours (unless you can, then go for it!), but you do need a pocket of peace each day. Protect that time. Guard it fiercely. It's where you refill your tank. Your well-being is not a luxury; it's the foundation that allows you to keep giving. When you care for yourself, you expand your capacity to care for others.

Day 184

Where can you find your tribe? Church, social groups, school, or parents of your children's friends.

You're not meant to do this alone. Your tribe is out there; people who get it, who've walked similar roads, who will sit beside you without trying to fix everything. Look toward your local community: church members, school groups, neighbors, or even online spaces. Sometimes your tribe isn't who you expect, but they show up at just the right time. And when you find them, you'll wonder how you ever did it without them. A caregiver with a circle of support is a caregiver with a lifeline. Find yours, nurture it, and lean into it often.

Day 185

Be open about your frustrations.

Bottling up frustration may feel noble, but it's not sustainable. You're allowed to say, "This is hard." You're allowed to say, "I'm frustrated." That doesn't mean you're failing; it means you're feeling. And when you speak your truth, others can respond with theirs. Someone out there has walked this road and might have wisdom you haven't heard yet. You don't have to vent to the whole world but find someone safe. A friend. A forum. A therapist. Don't carry this weight alone. Share the struggle. Be honest. Vulnerability isn't weakness, it's connection. And connection is what carries us through. Your words can lighten not only your load, but someone else's too. Sometimes the simple act of speaking out is the first step toward healing.

Day 186

Don't be afraid to let people help.

Help isn't a handout—it's a hand up. Letting someone do the dishes or run an errand doesn't make you less capable. It makes you smart. You cannot give endlessly without rest. That's not compassion, it's combustion. Allowing others to help creates space for you to breathe, heal, and remember who you are. You deserve time to rest, recharge, and reconnect with yourself. Care for yourself like you're someone worth helping—because you are. Don't wait for a breaking point. Let people step in before you fall out. Delegating care doesn't weaken your impact, it strengthens your sustainability.

Day 187

Let it hurt, then let it go

Pain is part of caregiving, whether it's grief over the changes you're witnessing, frustration with the demands, or the weight of exhaustion. Don't shove it down or pretend it's not there; let yourself feel it. Cry if you need to, talk it out, or simply acknowledge, *"This is hard."* But don't stay stuck in that pain. Once you've let it out, make the choice to release it, so it doesn't take up more space than it deserves. Letting go isn't about forgetting or ignoring; it's about freeing yourself to move forward with a clearer heart and mind. Each release creates room for peace, however small, to enter in. Over time, those moments of peace add up, reminding you that pain may visit, but it doesn't have to remain.

Day 188

Have some fun... you are allowed.

Caregiving can feel heavy, but joy isn't off-limits—you're allowed, and even encouraged, to have fun. Laughter and lightness are powerful medicines for both you and your loved one. Play their favorite music and sing along, share old photos and swap funny memories, or take a few minutes to watch a comedy show together. If they enjoy games, try a quick card game or puzzle. And when you have a quiet moment to yourself, do something that makes *you* smile; maybe read a lighthearted book, call a friend who makes you laugh, or step outside for fresh air. Fun doesn't erase the hard stuff, but it makes the journey lighter and more meaningful.

Day 189

Resource: Caringbridge.org

This site helps you keep friends and family updated without repeating the same tough conversations. With CaringBridge, you can create a private journal, share health updates, and allow others to leave messages of support. It's emotional relief for you and a lifeline for your support system. It's ideal when your time and energy are stretched thin, but you still want to keep people in the loop. Think of it as your caregiving command center meets love letter inbox. Easy, free, and surprisingly powerful.

Day 190

When you feel lost, reach out to friends
who can pull you out of your funk.

Caregiving can feel isolating, especially on the days when the weight of it all leaves you feeling stuck or lost. When you find yourself sinking into that heavy place, don't try to climb out alone. Reach out to the people who know how to find you, the ones who listen without judgment, who remind you who you are when you've forgotten. A simple text, a quick call, or even just sitting quietly with a trusted friend can shift the heaviness. You don't have to carry everything by yourself. Let the people who love you throw you a lifeline when you need it most. It's not weakness, it's wisdom.

Day 191

*Be thankful for the obvious miracles
and the hidden joys.*

Some blessings shout from the rooftops. Others whisper in the corner. Look for both. That moment of calm? That tiny smile? That warm cup of tea while the world rests? Those are gifts, too. Don't overlook them just because they're small. Gratitude isn't about perfection; it's about presence. When you pause to appreciate the glimmers, you train your heart to see beauty even on hard days. Miracles might not always be flashy. But they're there, tucked into daily life, waiting to be noticed. Choose to see them, name them, and let them lift you.

Day 192

Give yourself some grace and celebrate success.

Caregiving is tough, and you won't get everything perfect—and that's okay. Give yourself some grace for the moments that don't go as planned, and take time to acknowledge the wins, no matter how small they seem. Maybe it's managing a difficult day with patience, making your loved one smile, or simply showing up when you're exhausted. These moments matter and deserve to be celebrated. Don't wait for big milestones to feel proud—recognize the everyday victories that prove your strength and heart are showing up where it counts.

Day 193

People will never forget how you made them feel.

In caregiving, the way you make someone feel often speaks louder than the tasks you complete. Your tone of voice, your patience, and your kindness all leave a lasting imprint long after the details of the day are forgotten. A gentle touch, a shared laugh, or a moment of quiet understanding can turn an ordinary day into something meaningful. People may not remember every word you said or every task you handled, but they will remember how safe, loved, and cared for they felt in your presence. That's the legacy of true caregiving. It's a legacy that outlives the moment and lingers in the heart. And in the end, those feelings of love and safety are what matter most.

Day 194

You are somebody's reason to smile.

It might be the way you hum while folding laundry, your ridiculous dance moves in the kitchen, or your unwavering patience during hard days—but trust this: someone smiles because of you. Your presence brings light. Your kindness ripples out farther than you know. You don't have to be loud, flashy, or funny on cue—just being authentically you is enough to brighten someone's day. Never doubt your impact. You matter more than you realize, especially when you're just being real. So, keep showing up and sharing your light. Even on tough days, you're giving someone a reason to smile. And sometimes, that small spark you share is exactly what keeps another person going.

Day 195

Make time for yourself.

Caregiving demands so much of your energy and heart that without intentional breaks, you risk burning out. Even small moments matter, like sipping coffee in peace, taking a walk, reading a few pages of a book, or calling a friend just to chat. These pockets of time refill your tank and help you show up with patience and strength. When you care for yourself, you're not taking away from your loved one; you're ensuring you have the energy to keep caring well. Protect that time like it's essential, because it is. Think of it as tending the roots so the branches can keep reaching. A nourished caregiver is the best gift you can give.

Day 196

Stay true to your inner knowing.

Your gut has guided you through more than you realize. It's the quiet voice that says "yes," "no," or "not yet"—even when the noise around you is loud. Trust it. Others may second-guess your choices, but they don't live your life. Instincts are wisdom formed by experience, intuition, and love. Please don't ignore them. You don't need permission to trust yourself. Check facts but also check your spirit. If something feels off, pause. If it feels right, lean in. You were given those instincts for a reason. They are not guesses; they are guides. Listen closely. The more you honor that inner compass, the stronger it becomes. Over time, you'll find it leads you not just to the right choices, but to peace in making them.

Day 197

It's all shits and giggles until someone giggles and shits.

Welcome to the not-so-glamorous life of caregiving, where the absurd and the messy often waltz together. Sometimes, the only sane response is to laugh—and maybe light a candle for good measure. Humor isn't frivolous; it's grounding. It eases tension, cuts through the chaos, and proves that even the strangest moments can be survived. So, embrace the ridiculous. Let your dignity take a short break if it has to. A solid sense of humor is just as essential as a sturdy pair of gloves. When everything goes sideways, search for the funny. Because if you don't laugh... you'll probably cry. And honestly, both are healing. The gift is knowing when to lean into each. Either way, you're letting the weight out instead of keeping it bottled up.

Day 198

Read: The Conscious Caregiver: A Mindful Approach to Caring for Your Loved One Without Losing Yourself by Linda Abbit

This book is all about mindful caregiving; not just what you do, but how you are. Linda Abbit offers practical ways to stay grounded, present, and sane while caring for others. She tackles boundaries, self-talk, and burnout prevention without making you feel guilty. It's for anyone who tries to care deeply without losing themselves in the process. If you've ever felt like you're disappearing under the weight of your role, this book brings you back to center. It's like a wise mentor whispering, "You matter."

Day 199

Take care of yourself as if you were the most amazing person you've ever met.

Imagine if you treated yourself like someone you actually liked—someone whose needs mattered, whose time was valuable, and whose heart deserved protection. Wild, right? But you are that person. You've been showing up for others like a champ; now show up for yourself. Rest when you need to. Speak kindly to yourself. Do the thing that makes you feel alive again. You're not just "someone's caregiver," you are a whole human being, worthy of the same love and effort you give so freely. Don't just survive. Thrive. Care for yourself like you're someone who deserves joy. Because you do.

Day 200

What goes on a care calendar? Grocery runs, rides to appointments, childcare needs, pet care, socializing, house and yard maintenance, etc.

Don't carry it all in your head. A care calendar isn't just a planner, it's your permission to share the load. Document the recurring tasks: grocery runs, laundry, prescription pickups, transportation, pet feeding, social visits, yard work. Include self-care breaks for yourself. Then delegate. Let others choose what they can handle. When people say, "Let me know how I can help," this calendar becomes your response. You're not asking for favors, you're coordinating care. Let the calendar be your quiet teammate. You don't have to do it all. You just need to start sharing.

Day 201

When you are a primary caregiver, each day is a sprint.

From sunup to sundown, it can feel like you're in a constant race; meds, meals, emotions, and appointments all vying for your time. You hardly have a moment to breathe, let alone reflect. Even runners slow down between races. If every day feels like a full-speed dash, create tiny pauses for yourself. A deep breath. A stretch. A cup of tea you actually sit down to drink. You're running on love, but even love needs fuel. You can't win the caregiving marathon if you sprint yourself into the ground.

Day 202

Say to yourself, "This is good enough and
I'll make it better next time."

Perfection is exhausting, and originality can feel overrated on days when you're simply trying to survive. Give yourself permission to step back. You don't need to be brilliant, polished, or groundbreaking; you just need to be present. Some seasons are about steady maintenance, not dazzling reinvention. Tell yourself, "This will do for now. I'll revisit it with fresh eyes later." Choose progress over perfection. Choose peace over pressure. You're allowed to exhale and let "good enough" truly be enough. That's not laziness, it's wisdom. Let this be the year of enough, and if it still needs work next year? Great. No worries, you'll tackle it then. Life doesn't reward the most polished—it rewards the most persistent. And showing up, even imperfectly, is always more powerful than not showing up at all.

Day 203

*Learn from the mistakes of others. You can't live
long enough to make them all yourself."
— Eleanor Roosevelt*

Life's too short to learn everything the hard way. And in caregiving? Mistakes can be costly to your energy, your relationships, and your sanity. The good news? Other people have already blazed this trail, potholes and all. Read their stories and ask questions. Take the wisdom and skip the regret. Learning from others isn't cheating, it's smart. It's how we grow faster, suffer less, and make fewer emotional U-turns. You're not supposed to figure this out alone. Take notes from those who have stumbled and kept walking. They're handing you a flashlight. Use it. Let their lessons guide you forward.

Day 204

Done is better than perfect.

Done is better than perfect, especially in caregiving. You don't need to have everything flawlessly organized, every meal perfectly planned, or every detail executed without a hitch. What matters most is that your loved one feels cared for, safe, and supported, not that everything looks perfect on the outside. Perfection is exhausting and unrealistic, but progress, even in small steps, makes a real difference. Give yourself permission to let "good enough" be truly good enough. Your effort and heart are what count the most.

Day 205

If people want to help you, say YES!!!

You are not a one-person army. If someone offers help, let them. Don't block their blessing or yours by trying to be everything to everyone. The laundry doesn't care who folds it. The dishes don't judge. Say Yes. Accepting help isn't a sign of weakness; it's a smart move. It gives others a chance to love you in action, and it gives you precious breathing room. Repeat it: Yes. Let them vacuum, make a meal, cut the lawn, or run an errand. The world will keep turning, and you'll have more energy to give where it's most needed. Rest isn't earned only after you've done it all, it's part of sustaining yourself along the way. And by sharing the load, you're teaching others that care is a circle, not a solo act.

Day 206

It's OK to take a guilt-free break and leave your loved one in the care of a qualified person.

It's not just okay, but necessary to take a guilt-free break and let a trusted, qualified person step in. Caregiving is demanding, and trying to do it all on your own will only lead to burnout. Stepping away, even for a few hours, allows you to rest, reset, and come back with more patience and energy. Your loved one will benefit from your renewed strength, and you'll be reminded that it's okay to lean on others. Taking a break is part of sustainable, healthy caregiving. Think of it as maintenance for both body and soul; a pause that helps you keep going with steadiness instead of running on empty.

Day 207

Separate worries from concerns.

Not everything that makes your heart race deserves real estate in your mind. Some things are worries that are based on "what ifs" and fear. Others are concerns, grounded in facts and actionable next steps. Learn to tell the difference. Worry spins your wheels; concern helps you plan. Ask yourself: Can I do something about this? If yes, take a step. If not, take a breath. Worrying is like rocking in a chair—lots of movement with no forward motion. Concerns guide you; worries drain you. Name what's real, release what's not. Free up mental space for what matters. That's how peace begins—by sorting through the noise.

Day 208

Take care of yourself because you are no good to anyone when you're sick.

You can't pour from an empty cup let alone from a hospital bed. If you keep pushing yourself past exhaustion, your body will hit the brakes for you, and often at the worst time. Taking care of yourself is not indulgence—it's insurance. Sleep. Hydrate. Stretch. Laugh. Ask for help. Take the time now to tend to yourself, or your body will demand it later, and with interest. Caregivers are incredibly strong, but you're not indestructible. No one benefits when you're running on fumes. The healthiest version of you serves everyone better. Prioritize yourself like someone you're responsible for... because you are.

Day 209

*Take the words **always** and **never** out of your vocabulary.*

Absolutes are emotional traps. "I always mess up." "They never understand." Sound familiar? These words don't reflect reality; they reflect exhaustion, frustration, and a mind trying to make sense of the chaos. Replace them with truth: "This is hard right now." "Today was rough, but not every day is." Language shapes your mindset. Be kind with your words, especially the ones you speak to yourself. Life isn't black or white, it's layered, nuanced, and often gray with moments of gold. Drop the extremes. Make room for grace. Let your vocabulary leave space for change, growth, and second chances.

Day 210

Often, those who have been there, done that,
are the first to offer help.

Those who've walked the caregiving path often understand its weight better than anyone else, and they're usually the first to step up with help. They know the exhaustion, the emotional rollercoaster, and the moments when you just need someone to lighten the load. Don't hesitate to accept their offers, whether it's a meal, a listening ear, or a few hours of relief. Their support isn't just kindness; it's experience speaking, a quiet way of saying, "I know how hard this is, and you don't have to do it alone." Let their presence remind you that community is built one act of shared compassion at a time.

Day 211

Resource: Eldercare Locator
www.eldercare.acl.gov

This tool searches for you. You enter your location, and the Eldercare Locator connects you to local Area Agencies on Aging. These agencies often provide low- or no-cost services, such as transportation, caregiver training, legal aid, or respite care. It's federally supported, so the focus is on trusted, nonprofit resources—no junk or scams. It's especially valuable when you're caring for a loved one from a distance or are unfamiliar with their community. One search opens the door to dozens of lifelines, right in your backyard.

Day 212

All that matters is that you truly loved.

When the lists are done, the appointments are kept, and the days are behind you, what lasts? Love. Not the perfection of your care, but the heart behind it. Did you show up with kindness? Did you remain present during the challenging moments? Did you offer grace, laughter, and warmth? That's what they'll remember. And that's what you will carry forward. You won't regret not folding the towels just right, but you'll treasure the moments of love shared, even in the messy middle. Let love lead. Let it shape how you serve and how you live. That's the legacy that truly endures.

Day 213

"Anyone can hold the helm when the sea is calm."
— Publilius Syrus

It's easy to feel confident and capable when life is smooth and predictable, but caregiving rarely stays that way. The real test of your strength comes during the difficult moments, when plans fall apart, emotions run high, or unexpected challenges arise at your doorstep. Anyone can handle the easy days, but it's in the messy, exhausting, and uncertain times that your resilience truly shines. Those moments don't define your worth by how perfectly you handle them, but by your willingness to keep going, adapting, and showing up with heart even when it's hard.

Day 214

There's no greater value in life than caring for another.

There's no greater value in life than caring for another, because it's the purest form of love in action. Caregiving strips away all the unimportant things and reminds us of what truly matters: showing up, offering kindness, and being present for someone who needs you. It's not about grand gestures or perfection; it's about the countless small moments that add up to something deeply meaningful. When you care for someone, you give them dignity, comfort, and connection, and in return, you often discover a deeper sense of purpose within yourself. Few things leave a greater mark on the heart.

Day 215

Make an effort to stay well-connected with family and friends who can offer non-judgmental emotional support.

You don't need people who try to fix you. Instead, you need people who will sit with you. Stay close to those who offer understanding, not unsolicited advice. They might not be caregivers, but they care. Let them in. Share the highs and the lows. Don't isolate yourself in your strength. Connection is part of what keeps you grounded. Whether it's a quick check-in, a voice note, or a late-night meme, stay tethered. You're not meant to carry the emotional load alone. Support doesn't need to be loud or constant; it just needs to be real.

Day 216

Being happy means that you've decided to look beyond the imperfections.

Happiness isn't about a flawless life; it's about choosing to see the good, even in the middle of the mess. Perfection is an illusion; peace is a decision. When you shift your focus to gratitude, small joys, and meaningful moments, happiness finds you. It's not ignoring reality; it's adjusting your lens. The laundry will pile up, the to-do list will multiply, and things will go sideways. But amidst it all, laughter still exists. Love still shows up. Sunlight still spills across the floor. Perfection is rare, but contentment? That's available daily, if you choose to look for it.

Day 217

*Develop a forgiving attitude; most people
are doing the best they can.*

Developing a forgiving attitude can make caregiving and life so much lighter. Most people, whether it's family members, healthcare professionals, or even strangers offering advice, are doing the best they can with what they know. Misunderstandings, dropped balls, or unhelpful comments often stem from exhaustion or a lack of experience, rather than malice. Holding on to frustration only drains your energy and adds tension where it's not needed. When you can let go of minor mistakes and choose grace instead, you create space for understanding, better communication, and a calmer heart, for yourself and everyone around you.

Day 218

*Read: Can't We Talk About Something More Pleasant?
by Roz Chast*

Roz Chast's graphic memoir is refreshingly honest and often hilariously heartbreaking. She chronicles her parents' aging and decline with wit, frustration, and surprising tenderness. If you've ever laughed inappropriately at the absurdity of caregiving (or wanted to) this one's for you. Through cartoons and anecdotes, Chast reminds us that it's okay to be overwhelmed, to feel guilty, and to find humor in hard things. You'll nod, cry, and laugh your way through it. It's therapy in comic form.

Day 219

Expect to feel like quitting at least a dozen times.

No matter how passionate, loving, or committed you are, there will be days when you want to throw in the towel. That doesn't mean you're weak. It means you're human. Caregiving will stretch you, test you, and sometimes downright exhaust you. But expecting those moments of doubt helps you face them with grace. When they come, pause. Don't quit, rest. Breathe. Cry. Vent. Then remind yourself why you started, who you're doing this for, and what truly matters. The feeling of quitting will pass. Your strength will remain. And tomorrow? That towel you wanted to throw might just become your cape.

Day 220

Find freedom in the word No.

"No" isn't rejection, it's self-respect. It's a boundary. It's breathing room. Every time you say no to something that drains or overwhelms you, you say yes to rest, clarity, and sanity. You are not obligated to explain, justify, or apologize. You don't need to earn your peace by pleasing everyone else. "No" protects your energy for what matters most. Practice saying it gently, firmly, and without guilt. It's not a dirty word; it's a sacred one. Let it create space in your life where resentment once resided. You don't have to do it all. You have to do what's right for you.

Day 221

One day, everything clicks; the next day, nothing will.

Progress rarely moves in a straight line. Some days, you're a caregiving ninja—on time, on task, even sneaking in a moment to sip your tea while it's hot. Other days, it feels like your brain clocked out and forgot to tell you. That's normal. Life doesn't reward perfection; it rewards grit. The trick is not to measure your worth by your hardest moments. Celebrate the good days as victories, and see the rough ones as proof that you're still in the fight. Effort counts. You're not failing, you're human. The rhythm will return. Until then, breathe. Reset. Try again tomorrow. And when tomorrow comes, it carries a fresh chance to do a little better, or at least a little differently. Even the smallest step is still progress.

Day 222

Organize medical information so it's up to date and easy to find.

In emergencies and even routine checkups, clarity saves time and stress. Keep a binder, folder, or digital file of essential documents: medication lists, insurance cards, test results, allergies, and contact numbers. Update it regularly and store it in a location where others can access it if needed. Label it clearly. This isn't just about being "on top of things," it's about being prepared when the unexpected happens. You'll thank yourself later. So will your loved one. A little effort now prevents big headaches later. And honestly? It just feels good to flip through a binder and say, "I've got that right here."

Day 223

Get out of the house!!! Even if it's just for a walk around the block.

Sometimes, the best therapy is a walk on the sidewalk and some fresh air. When the walls feel like they're closing in, the dishes are mocking you, and your brain is overloaded, step outside for just a few minutes. Movement clears mental fog, fresh air resets your mood, and being outside reminds you that the world is still turning (even if your laundry isn't). You don't need a destination, just a few deep breaths and a change of scenery. Permit yourself to leave the chaos behind, if only for a walk around the block. Your sanity will thank you.

Day 224

Hardships often prepare ordinary people for an extraordinary destiny.

Life rarely hands out growth without a bit of grit. The struggle you're facing isn't proof that you're failing; it might be shaping you into someone stronger, wiser, and more compassionate. Extraordinary strength often rises from ordinary beginnings and difficult circumstances. You're being prepared, not punished. Every hard day is carving out a depth in you that joy alone can't reach. You don't have to love the process, but trust that something meaningful is being formed. You're becoming the version of yourself who will look back and say, "I made it. And I'm better because of it." This is the middle of your becoming.

Day 225

Do something for the kid in you every day.

The grown-up version of you may be handling medications, bills, and emotional landmines, but inside, there's still a kid who wants to play. Nurture that inner child. Eat a popsicle. Dance to cheesy music. Draw with sidewalk chalk or watch cartoons guilt-free. These moments aren't frivolous; they're healing. That playful energy reminds you of joy, curiosity, and lightness; all things caregiving can drain. Reconnect with wonder, even briefly. It's not childish; it's soul care. Your inner kid deserves attention, laughter, and the chance to exist outside the seriousness of it all. Feed her. Honor him. Let that spark of fun keep you lit.

Day 226

Look in the mirror and say something encouraging to yourself every day.

You speak kindness to everyone else—now it's time to speak it to yourself. Look yourself in the eyes and say something true, something kind, something hopeful. "You're strong." "You're doing great." "You made it through another hard day." Affirmations aren't just cheesy sayings—they rewire your inner dialogue. Your reflection is more than tired eyes and messy hair; it's the face of someone who keeps showing up. Someone worthy of encouragement. Make it a habit. Say it out loud. Let your voice be the one cheering you on. Because you deserve to hear from your biggest advocate... you.

Day 227

Don't wait for the moment to become a memory.

In the moment, it's just another Tuesday. But later? That quick laugh, that quiet smile, or that shared silence becomes a treasure. Caregiving is full of tiny, ordinary moments that don't seem like much... until they're gone. Pay attention. Hold space. You don't need grand gestures to create meaning. Sometimes it's in the way you hand over a glass of water or gently tuck someone in. These small acts become sacred over time. Be present, not perfect. One day, you'll look back and realize how much love was packed into those tiny, forgettable seconds. Those are the real gold.

Day 228

Success consists of a series of little daily victories.

Forget the finish line—let's talk about the little wins. The moment you stayed calm. The snack finally eaten. The paperwork filed. The deep breath instead of a meltdown. These are victories, and they count. Success isn't always shiny or public. Sometimes it looks like showing up when you wanted to hide or keeping your cool when you were one eye twitch away from losing it. Celebrate those moments. They're not small, they're sacred. Your day isn't measured by perfection, but by perseverance. Stack those small wins. That's how mountains move: one pebble, one choice, one deep breath at a time. And with each small step, you're proving to yourself that you're stronger than the struggle.

Day 229

*To the world, you might be one person, but
to one person, you might be the world.*

You may not be in the spotlight. You may not get applause. But to someone, you are everything. You're the steady presence. The comforting hand. The one who shows up again and again when it's hard, inconvenient, or thankless. You are a home base, a safety net, and a warm hug rolled into one. Never underestimate the power of your presence. The world may not notice, but that one person sees you as their anchor. And in this wild life, that kind of love matters more than titles, trophies, or trending hashtags. You're someone's whole world—and that makes you extraordinary.

Day 230

*When we give ourselves compassion, we are opening
our hearts in a way that can transform our lives.*

We are often our harshest critics. But what if you spoke to yourself the way you would to someone you love? What if you forgave yourself for the forgotten appointment, the short fuse, the tears? That shift from judgment to grace is life-changing. Compassion softens the hard days, lightens the shame, and reminds you: you are enough, as you are, even now. When you open your heart inward, the overflow outward becomes more powerful. Start with kindness to yourself. The ripple effect? Peace. Clarity. Healing. Give yourself the grace you'd give to anyone else. You're not just worthy; you're wired for compassion.

Day 231

You don't always need a plan.

Life loves to throw curveballs, and sometimes your color-coded plan won't survive the first pitch. That's okay. When things feel uncertain, pause. Breathe. Let go of the need to control every twist. Trust that the next step will reveal itself when you're ready. You don't need to have it all figured out to move forward. Some of the best breakthroughs come from surrender, not strategy. You can't map everything, but you can choose calm, openness, and faith. Let today unfold without gripping too tightly. You may be surprised by how beautifully things align when you breathe and let life flow.

Day 232

If you can do little things well, trust that you can do bigger things too.

If you can handle the little things with care and intention, trust that you have what it takes to tackle the bigger challenges, too. Caregiving is built on small, consistent acts such as organizing medications, preparing meals, offering comfort, and each one strengthens your confidence and resilience. Those everyday wins are proof that you're capable, resourceful, and stronger than you realize. When bigger tasks or more challenging moments come along, remember the foundation you've already built. The same skills, patience, and heart that guide you through the small things will carry you through the big ones.

Day 233

Executive ability is deciding quickly and getting somebody else to do the work.

Leadership isn't about doing it all; it's about knowing what needs doing and who can do it best. Delegate like a boss. You don't need to control every detail to be competent. True executive ability is choosing wisely, acting swiftly, and trusting others to handle it from there. Yes, even the laundry. Especially the laundry. Caregivers often feel pressure to manage every aspect, but a strategic approach beats burnout. Be decisive. Be smart. Be the one who says, "You take this; I'll take that," and then actually lets go. That's not lazy, that's legendary.

Day 234

Make sure you're getting enough sleep.

Sleep isn't optional. It's essential. And no, surviving on caffeine and sheer willpower doesn't count as a superpower; it's a one-way ticket to burnout. Your brain needs rest. Your body needs recovery. And your heart? It requires quiet time to heal from the emotional weight you carry. Sure, there's always more to do, but you'll do better with rest. Protect your sleep as if it were sacred. Turn off the screens. Ask for help. Say no to one more thing. A well-rested you is a calmer, kinder, and more capable you. Sleep isn't selfish, it's smart. Prioritize it. Your future self will thank you.

Day 235

Today, do as YOU please.

Today, give yourself permission to do something that's just for *you*. Caregiving often puts everyone else's needs first, but you deserve moments that bring joy, peace, or even a little indulgence. Whether it's taking a quiet walk, reading a book, enjoying your favorite treat, or simply resting without guilt, let today include something that brings you pleasure. These small acts of self-kindness aren't selfish; they're how you refill your energy and remember that your life matters too.

Day 236

You are a part of a puzzle in someone's life. You may never know where you fit, but someone's life may never be complete without you in it.

You don't always get to see the full picture, but trust this: you matter. In someone's life, your presence makes things whole. Maybe it's the way you listen, how you show up, or the simple comfort of your laugh. You're a piece of someone's life. Just like a puzzle isn't complete without every piece, someone's life is not complete without you. You don't need to be the center to be essential. Even when it feels like your contributions are small or invisible, they're forming something beautiful. Keep showing up, even when you don't know why. You're someone's missing puzzle piece, and they're grateful you exist.

Day 237

Resource: Family Caregiver Alliance
www.caregiver.org

If you want to feel understood and equipped, FCA is your new best friend. This resource hub offers educational materials, online support groups, interactive tools, and even state-by-state legal guides. Their content is practical but deeply empathetic, especially when you're feeling emotionally stretched or lost. FCA also supports caregivers of people with brain disorders, including Alzheimer's, stroke, and Parkinson's. Their CareNav tool is particularly helpful for getting a tailored care roadmap. This isn't just a website, it's a support system that knows what you're going through and wants to make it lighter.

Day 238

You can't be detached and effective.

Caregiving is personal—messy, emotional, heart-wide-open personal. And that's a good thing. You can't numb yourself and still connect. You can't wall off your heart and expect to care well. Detachment might feel like protection, but it also blocks presence, empathy, and impact. Your effectiveness depends on your ability to engage, to feel, and to respond with your full humanity. Yes, it's risky. Yes, it's draining. But being fully present is what changes lives—yours included. So don't fear feeling. Let it ground you, guide you, and make your caregiving real. That's where the magic happens: when you choose to stay soft in a hard world.

Day 239

Work hard for things that matter to you.

Not everything deserves your energy, but the things that truly matter? Fight for them. In caregiving, your days are filled with choices, and it's easy to get lost in the noise of what *should* get done. But when you focus your time and heart on what *actually* matters to you, whether that's quality time with your loved one, protecting your peace, or honoring a promise, you'll find strength you didn't know you had. Working hard is noble, but working hard for what you care deeply about? That's purpose. Let that guide and fuel you. Everything else can wait.

Day 240

The sooner you realize that doing it all is unattainable, the more peaceful your moments will be.

Repeat after me: "I can't do it all." Say it again, slower. Let it sink in. You were never meant to do everything, fix everything, or be everything to everyone. That's not noble, it's unsustainable. Give yourself the freedom to let some things go. Imperfectly done is still done. Breathe. Prioritize. Delegate. Rest. You'll be amazed how peace sneaks in once you stop clinging to the myth of doing it all. You don't need to hustle for worthiness. You're already enough. Your presence is more powerful than your perfection. Let that be the new goal: peace over perfection, presence over performance.

Day 241

Permit yourself to make mistakes.

You're going to mess up. You'll forget something, snap when you're tired, or drop a ball you were certain you could juggle. And that's okay. Mistakes aren't the enemy; shame is. Give yourself permission to be human. Learn from the slip-ups. Laugh when you can. Apologize when needed. Then keep moving forward. Caregiving isn't a test you ace with a perfect score, it's a journey of love, learning, and showing up even when it's hard. Mistakes don't define you; how you respond to them does. Let them teach you, not torment you. You're not a robot. You're a real person doing real work in real time. Grace belongs in this process just as much as effort. And often, the imperfect moments become the ones filled with the most love.

Day 242

Strength comes from overcoming the things you once thought you couldn't.

Real strength isn't loud or flashy, it's quiet persistence in the face of doubt. It's doing the thing you thought might break you. It's standing back up after the fall. You gain strength not by lifting the easy stuff, but by pushing through what feels impossible. You're stronger now than you were last month. Stronger than yesterday. Not because life got easier, but because you grew. Celebrate that. The things you once feared? You're facing them now. That's growth. That's grit. That strength will carry you through caregiving, through life, and through every challenge that's still ahead.

Day 243

When someone asks how you are doing,
it's Ok to be honest.

You don't have to wear the "I'm fine" mask all the time. When someone asks, be real. You can say, "It's been a tough week," or "I'm exhausted, but hanging in there." Vulnerability isn't weakness; it's honesty. And it creates a connection. You're not burdening anyone—you're opening a door to deeper support. Let people meet the real you, not the curated version. Because in those honest moments, friendships deepen, support strengthens, and healing begins. You're allowed to tell the truth, even if it's messy. The right people won't run from your truth; they'll lean in closer. And those are the people who remind you that you're never truly alone in this.

Day 244

Find a practice that calms your mind.
Perhaps yoga, tai chi, or meditation.

Your mind needs peace just as much as your schedule needs structure. Whether it's yoga, tai chi, meditation, prayer, or simply sitting quietly with your coffee, find a rhythm that restores your calm. You don't need to be perfect at it; you just need to show up for yourself. These practices teach you how to breathe when life feels like it's holding you under. It's not about escaping reality; it's about grounding yourself in it. Make space for stillness. Let calm become your superpower. And remember, peace doesn't scream for your attention; it waits quietly until you come looking for it.

Day 245

---

*Organizing and automating medications
can be a true timesaver.*

Organizing and automating medications can save you countless hours and stress. Simple steps, such as requesting a 90-day supply, setting up mail-order or auto-delivery with the pharmacy, and syncing refill dates, can eliminate those last-minute pharmacy runs. Pill organizers or color-coded pillboxes can help track daily doses, while medication reminder apps or alarms on your phone ensure nothing is missed. Some caregivers even use a checklist on the fridge or a shared digital calendar with family members to stay on track. The more you can automate and simplify this process, the more mental energy you free up for the other parts of caregiving that truly need your attention.

Day 246

Compassion is best shown through action.

Compassion isn't something you simply feel; it's something you do. It's the meal you drop off when someone's too tired to cook, the quiet hand you hold when there are no words, the moments you stay present even when it's uncomfortable. True compassion crosses every barrier—cultural, emotional, and spiritual—because it's rooted in genuine care. In caregiving, compassion becomes part of your everyday language, expressed through patience, small acts of service, and the time you willingly give. It doesn't need an audience or recognition to matter. Often, it's the smallest, simplest gestures offered with big love that leave the deepest mark.

Day 247

It's OK not to be OK.

It's okay not to be okay... really. Caregiving can be overwhelming, and expecting yourself to stay strong every moment isn't realistic or fair. Some days will break you open with exhaustion or emotion, and that doesn't mean you're failing; it means you're human. Allow yourself to feel what you feel. Cry if you need to, rest when you can, and lean on others for support. You don't have to carry it all perfectly. Admitting you're not okay is often the first step to finding the help, healing, or relief you need. Strength isn't about never falling apart—it's about allowing yourself to be real and still choosing to keep going. And every time you rise again, you prove that not being okay is only part of the story, not the ending.

Day 248

A kind gesture can reach a wound that only compassion can heal.

Sometimes words fall short, but kindness? It always lands. A warm glance, a soft tone, a thoughtful note; these small things carry tremendous healing power. You never know what silent pain someone is holding. Your kindness may be the only grace they experience today. And it works both ways: giving kindness soothes your soul, too. It reconnects you with your humanity. Compassion doesn't need credentials. It just needs intention. Be generous with it. Let kindness be the language you speak when there's nothing else to say. It won't fix everything, but it will always help. That's the magic of empathy.

Day 249

Accept what you cannot change.

Some things are simply out of your hands; timelines, diagnoses, other people's choices. You can fight the unchangeable or make peace with it. Acceptance doesn't mean giving up. It means shifting your focus to what is within your control: your attitude, your actions, your boundaries. It's okay to grieve what you can't change. But then, let go. Holding on will only exhaust you. There is strength in surrender—not to circumstance, but to wisdom. Save your energy for the things that can grow, heal, and evolve. Acceptance isn't passive; it's powerful. And it creates room for peace where resistance once lived.

Day 250

When the day is busy and the workload unbearable, someone says or does something, and you know you've made a difference in their life.

In the whirlwind of to-do lists and caregiving chaos, it's easy to miss the magic. But every now and then, someone looks at you with gratitude, says "thank you," or smiles just a little softer, and in that moment, you know that you matter. Your care is changing something. It may not be flashy or widely praised, but it's real. Those small moments are everything. Let them anchor you on hard days. Let them remind you why you keep showing up. You are making a difference, whether you hear it every day or not. And that difference is beautiful.

Day 251

Appreciate how special it is to care for others.

Caregiving isn't just work—it's an act of love in motion. Yes, it's hard. Yes, it's messy. But there's something deeply sacred about being the one who shows up. You're part of life's most meaningful moments, offering comfort, presence, and dignity when it's needed most. Not everyone gets to do that. Don't let the chaos or fatigue blind you to the beauty in it. You're making someone's life easier, lighter, and safer. Pause to breathe and recognize what a gift it is to be a giver of care. You're doing something extraordinary. Don't forget that.

Day 252

Compassion for others begins with kindness to ourselves.

You can't pour from a cup that's full of self-judgment. Genuine compassion starts inward, with gentleness toward your own heart, especially when you feel like you're falling short. When you treat yourself with kindness, your capacity to care for others expands. So, talk to yourself like you would someone you love. Forgive yourself. Nourish yourself. Encourage yourself. Because caregiving doesn't require perfection, it requires presence. And the more you offer yourself grace, the more grace you'll have to give. Self-kindness isn't indulgent; it's foundational. Be soft with yourself first. Everything else flows from there.

Day 253

Ask about medical assistance at every doctor's visit.

Medical needs evolve faster than you think. What wasn't necessary a month ago may now be essential. Every appointment is an opportunity to reassess both the patient's needs and your own as the caregiver. Inquire about available resources, support services, programs, and new opportunities. Don't assume they'll volunteer the info. You may have to advocate for it. Bring a list and ask the "what ifs." You're not being annoying, you're being thorough. It's easier to plan ahead than play catch-up. Care is a moving target, and questions are your best tools. Speak up, stay curious, and treat each visit like a mini strategy session.

Day 254

You are not meant to do-all or be-all.

You're not a superhero, you're human. And even superheroes have backup. Ask for help. Not when you're on the edge, but now. Whether it's meals, errands, respite care, or just someone to sit with you while you cry, your support system needs an invitation. Please don't wait for people to guess what you need help with; they probably don't know how to offer. Speak it plainly: "I need help." It doesn't make you weak. It makes you smart, resourceful, and honest. You're not meant to carry it all. Let others lend their strength. And when they do? Receive it with open arms and zero guilt. Help is not an extravagance; it's a lifeline. Every time you accept it, you are reminded that caregiving was never meant to be a solo act.

Day 255

*Allow your loved one to continue doing as much
as they can for themselves.*

Allowing your loved one to do as much as they can for themselves is practical and empowering. Even small tasks, such as brushing their hair, choosing their clothes, or preparing part of a meal, can help them maintain independence and dignity. It might take longer, and it might be tempting to step in and "just get it done," but letting them stay involved in their own care helps preserve their confidence and sense of purpose. Your role isn't to do everything for them, but to support them in doing what they're still able to do. This balance not only strengthens their spirit but also lightens your load in meaningful ways.

Day 256

*Resource: National Respite Locator Service
www.archrespite.org*

Everyone needs a break, and this tool helps you find one. The National Respite Locator enables you to locate temporary care providers in your area so that you can step away without guilt. Whether you need a few hours to recharge or a weekend for self-care, this service connects you with vetted respite programs and providers. Respite isn't optional; it's a necessity for sustainable caregiving. This tool is your permission slip to rest. And the best part? It's built by people who understand how hard it is to even ask for help.

Day 257

*Be in the moment with them. They may not
remember you are there, but YOU do.*

Presence is a gift, even if it goes unnoticed. When memory fades, conversation falters, or awareness dims, your time still matters. They may not recall your words, but they feel your warmth. They may forget the moment, but your love leaves a mark. And you will remember the hand you held, the smile you caught, or the quiet breath between you. Being fully present isn't about being seen, it's about seeing. This is where connection lives; in the now. Stay there. Be there. That moment may vanish for them, but it becomes part of your forever. And that is beautiful.

Day 258

*When researching care facilities, look for those that share
values that align with yours and your loved ones.*

Not every facility is the right fit. Beyond cost and location, ask more profound questions: Do their values align with yours? Do they honor autonomy, compassion, culture, and faith? How do they address emotional care, in addition to physical needs? Take a tour of the space and observe how the staff interacts with residents. Inquire about staff turnover, activity options, meal arrangements, and visiting hours. Your loved one's dignity deserves more than convenience; it deserves alignment. Trust yourself. Ask tough questions. Because you're not just choosing a place, you're choosing a partner in care.

Day 259

Being a caregiver will severely impact your lifestyle.

Caregiving doesn't just add tasks, it redefines life. Your routines, personal time, and relationships will shift. It's okay to grieve the "old normal" while learning to embrace the new one. You're not doing anything wrong; you're just living a life that demands more flexibility, patience, and heart. Let go of the expectation that things will ever return exactly as they were. This is your new rhythm. It may not be what you chose, but it can still hold meaning, growth, and even joy. Adjust your pace. Redefine success. And remember, even in this new normal, you are still your own person.

Day 260

There is strength in accepting help.

Let someone bring dinner, fold laundry, and sit with your loved one for a quiet evening. Accepting help doesn't mean you are not capable; it means you're wise enough not to do it alone. You're not proving anything by running yourself into the ground. Let go of the superhero myth. Real strength knows when to say, "Yes, I could use that." Let people show up for you. Let them serve you with the same love you offer others. Accepting help doesn't diminish you; it honors your humanity. And you're allowed to be human. You don't lose dignity when you lean on others; you gain endurance. And in that shared care, both you and your loved one are better held.

Day 261

*Believe that you are doing the best you can and making
the best decisions possible at any given time.*

Self-doubt is loud, but truth is gentler. And here's the truth: you're doing the best you can with the knowledge, resources, and emotional bandwidth you have right now. Every choice is made with love, even when it's complicated or imperfect. Don't judge yourself by hindsight—give yourself the grace of context. You're navigating uncharted territory. There's no playbook for this. Trust your heart. Trust that even on the messiest days, your care matters. Just presence and intention, not perfection. Keep choosing with compassion. And when in doubt? Remind yourself: doing your best is more than enough.

Day 262

*Break large tasks into smaller steps that you
can do one at a time.*

Overwhelm loves a long list. Don't let it win. When a task feels massive, break it down. What's the very first step? Just do that. Then the next. You don't have to conquer the mountain; you have to take the next breath, the next call, the next paper off the pile. Momentum builds quietly. Checking off small steps creates clarity and confidence. And if today only allows for one of those steps? That's still progress. You're not behind; you're pacing yourself. One task, one moment, one choice at a time. That's how caregiving works. Forward is forward, no matter the speed.

Day 263

Sometimes the person who's been there for everyone else needs someone there for them.

I see you—the rock, the helper, the one everyone leans on. But I also see your tired heart, the quiet moments when you wonder if you can keep going. It's okay to fall apart a little. It's okay to let someone wrap you in the same care and compassion you give so freely. Being strong doesn't mean holding every burden alone; it means knowing when to say, "I need you." You don't have to do this by yourself. You're not alone, and you never were.

Day 264

By loving yourself more, you love the person you are caring for more.

Your well-being is the foundation of your caregiving. When you treat yourself with kindness, rest, and compassion, you show up more fully for others. Self-love isn't selfish; it's strategic. When your tank is full, you respond with more patience, clarity, and grace. When it's empty, even the simplest requests can feel like burdens. The person you're caring for benefits most when you take care of yourself, too. So, nourish your soul, protect your peace, and say yes to things that restore you. Your love for them grows stronger when it's rooted in love for yourself. Refill to overflow. That's the secret.

Day 265

---

*Read: Living with Dying by Jahnna Beecham
and Katie Ortlip*

This book is the friend you need when death is part of the caregiving equation. Written by a hospice nurse and a family caregiver, it's compassionate, practical, and beautifully clear. It demystifies end-of-life care with wisdom and grace. From tough conversations to comfort care, it walks beside you without judgment or fear. If you're navigating anticipatory grief or preparing to say goodbye, this book offers the kind of comfort that feels both deeply human and fiercely informed.

Day 266

---

*During the end-of-life care phase, let medical
professionals take the lead with caregiving.*

Hospice care as your loved one nears the end of their life can be a gift for both you and your loved one, so let the medical professionals take the lead with hands-on caregiving. Nurses, aides, and hospice teams are trained to handle the physical care, which allows you to step out of the "doing" and into simply *being* with your loved one. This shift can help prevent resentment or exhaustion from building up, freeing you to focus on what matters most in those final moments: sharing memories, telling stories, holding their hand, or sitting in peaceful silence. Sometimes, the greatest act of love is letting go of the tasks so you can just *love them.* In the end, it's presence, not perfection, that becomes the most precious gift.

Day 267

Encourage visitors, but remember boundaries.

Visitors can be a gift, but for someone who's ill or tired, extended visits can feel overwhelming. Encourage friends and family to visit, but set clear expectations by sharing which days and times work best. Also, gently suggest that they keep visits brief. Choose an amount of time that allows for connection without causing exhaustion. That's often enough to brighten someone's day without exhausting them. Let people know it's about quality, not quantity. A warm chat, a shared laugh, or simply sitting together can mean more than hours of conversation. When visitors respect the person's energy and routine, everyone leaves feeling lighter and more connected.

Day 268

There is no cookie-cutter formula for caregiving.

Don't compare your caregiving journey to someone else's. Every situation has its twists, personalities, and emotional weather. What worked for your neighbor might flop for you. That's not failure, it's reality. Your path is valid, even if it's messy or unconventional. You're not doing it wrong. You're doing what's right for your loved one, with the tools you have. That's enough. Give yourself permission to adapt, adjust, and abandon what doesn't serve. You're not building a perfect blueprint; you're creating something far more personal—a bridge of love, one step at a time.

Day 269

Honor your loved one's wishes, but know those decisions might not be popular.

Honoring your loved one's wishes can be one of the hardest—and most important—parts of caregiving. Their choices about treatment, medication, or end-of-life care might not sit well with everyone in the family, but it's not about pleasing the crowd, it's about respecting *them*. You may find yourself in the middle of emotional disagreements or feeling judged for supporting their decisions, but staying true to their wishes is an act of love and integrity. It's not easy, but it's what they deserve: to have their voice heard, even when others might not agree.

Day 270

Sometimes you have to say, "We do better when we work together."

Caregivers and their loved ones won't always see eye to eye, and that's normal. Tension can surface when independence meets assistance, or when frustration bubbles up on both sides. Instead of forcing your way through a disagreement, pause and acknowledge the challenge. A simple, "I know this is hard for both of us," can ease the tension and open the door to working together. Collaboration, such as asking for their input, offering choices, and finding middle ground, can turn a standoff into a partnership. You don't have to have all the answers; sometimes the best solution is found together. When you meet each other with patience instead of pressure, caregiving becomes less of a battle and more of a bond.

Day 271

*Caregiving isn't just about tasks –
it's also about relationships.*

Sure, the to-do list is long: meds, meals, appointments, but underneath it all, caregiving is relational. It's about connection, presence, and love expressed through the simplest acts. It's eye contact. A shared joke. A reassuring touch. These moments build a bridge between you and the one you're caring for. Don't let the tasks eclipse the person. Let yourself slow down enough to see your loved one. Even when memory fades or words are few, the relationship remains. Nurture it. Let it soften the rough days. The tasks will blur with time, but the relationship is the part that will stay with you forever.

Day 272

Boundaries are crucial for both of you.

Boundaries aren't walls; they're welcome mats with limits. They create safety, clarity, and respect. Whether it's quiet hours, scheduled breaks, or personal space, boundaries help you avoid resentment and burnout. They teach your loved one what to expect, and they remind you that you're allowed to have space and structure. Be clear. Be kind. Be consistent. You're not doing anyone any favors by saying yes to everything. Ground rules protect relationships by giving everyone room to breathe. Don't be afraid to set them. Placing a boundary today prevents a meltdown tomorrow. Boundaries may feel hard at first, but they often become the very thing that keeps you going

Day 273

Resource: The National Alliance for Caregiving

This organization is leading the charge on caregiving awareness, research, and policy. They advocate for caregivers at the national level and provide free reports, tools, and connections to other major caregiver networks. If you're feeling like the system wasn't built for you, this is the group working to change that. Their studies help shape legislation and workplace policies that make life easier for caregivers. You'll also find real-world stories, webinars, and thought-provoking resources that validate the challenges you face daily. Advocacy meets empathy here.

Day 274

When they're ready to talk, listen.

Listen—even when the conversation feels uncomfortable. If your loved one wants to talk about end-of-life care, funeral wishes, or other difficult topics, resist the urge to change the subject or shut it down. These are their wishes, their voice, and their chance to be heard. Lean in, take notes, and honor the courage it takes for them to share. You don't have to have all the answers; you just need to be present. Sometimes the greatest gift you can give is simply to listen, even when your heart wants to run the other way. Your willingness to stay says, "You matter, and your words matter." And later, you'll carry comfort in knowing you honored their truth instead of avoiding it.

Day 275

*Self-care suggestion: stretch for at least five minutes
every day, prioritizing your back and hips.*

Your body holds tension in places you don't even realize, until it starts shouting back. Daily stretching keeps you flexible, balanced, and less prone to injury. Caregiving involves repetitive movements, awkward lifting, and constant motion. Focus on your back and hips, which are your power centers. Take five minutes when you wake up or before bed. YouTube is full of quick stretch routines. Or touch your toes, twist gently, and breathe. This small ritual can prevent significant pain. Make it non-negotiable.

Day 276

Come to terms with feeling overwhelmed (it will happen).

Overwhelm is a natural side effect of caregiving. It means you care deeply and you're doing a lot. But you don't have to say yes to everything. It's okay to set limits. In fact, it's essential. Be honest with yourself. What can you really handle right now? What needs to wait, or be shared? Draw those boundaries, and guard them like your peace depends on it (because it does). Saying no doesn't mean you don't care. It means you're choosing what matters most and making sure you don't burn out while trying to save everyone else. Remember, the people who truly love you would rather hear "no" than watch you collapse under the weight of too much. Protecting your capacity today ensures you'll still have the strength to show up tomorrow. And that's how caregiving becomes sustainable instead of overwhelming.

Day 277

True compassion shifts everything.

True compassion turns tasks into connection and people into souls. When you care with open eyes and an open heart, you stop seeing people as interruptions—and start seeing them as fellow travelers. That doesn't mean you never get tired (you will), but it does mean you begin to understand each moment as an invitation to relate, not just react. Compassion says, "We're in this together," even when the going gets heavy. And ironically? The more compassion you give, the more energy you often receive, because you're connecting, not just coping. That's where the beauty of caregiving begins.

Day 278

*Connect with other people and families
in a similar situation.*

There's power in "Me too." Other caregivers understand your exhaustion, your questions, your fears because they're living it, too. Join a support group, attend a local gathering, or find an online forum. You don't have to navigate this alone. Shared stories lead to shared strength. Sometimes, just knowing that someone else understands is enough to make the next day bearable. Connections don't have to be deep or daily; they just have to be real. Community makes the caregiving road feel less lonely. And sometimes, it gives you more than support; it gives you lifelong friendships forged in the fire.

Day 279

Two great resources: The Office of the Aging and the Administration on Aging.

You don't have to guess where to find support. The Eldercare Locator is a powerful resource that connects you to your local Area Agency on Aging. Need help with meals, respite care, home modifications, or caregiver training? They can guide you. The services are often free or low-cost and are made just for people like you. Don't let pride, confusion, or the overwhelm of options stop you. One phone call could unlock real relief. You're not alone in this. There are programs designed to help you help your loved one.

Day 280

Always ask what resources are available.

New programs. Discounted services. Free supplies. Helpful apps. Support groups. Grants. Caregiver coaching. There's more available than you probably realize, but you won't find it if you don't ask. Make it a habit to regularly check for updates and opportunities. Talk to your doctor, local library, church, or a support group about what's out there. The internet is your ally, too. Resources evolve, new ones emerge, and far too many go unused simply because no one knows about them. Stay curious, stay vocal, and stay resourceful. Help is out there, and often, it's just one bold question away. Keep a running list of what you discover, because what you don't need today might be exactly what you need tomorrow. And when you share those resources with others, you multiply the support far beyond yourself.

Day 281

Resource: Veteran Directed Care Program; a program designed for veterans who need daily assistance.

This program provides veterans with the opportunity to receive daily assistance on their own terms. If your loved one served in the military and needs help at home, this service lets them direct their own care. They may even hire a trusted family member or friend. It's not just about aid; it's about autonomy. Veterans get a say in how, when, and by whom they're cared for. It's a beautiful blend of respect, dignity, and practicality. Connect with your local VA to explore this underutilized but life-changing program.

Day 282

If you work outside the home and you're a caregiver, consider taking a short-term leave.

You're juggling more than one full-time job, and burnout isn't just possible; it's inevitable if you never step back. If your employer offers short-term leave, or if you qualify for the Family and Medical Leave Act (FMLA), which protects your job while you take unpaid leave, explore those options before you reach a breaking point. Caregiving demands your full heart and focus, but you can't give your best when you're running on empty. Your job will still be there, but your health and well-being won't wait. Advocate for yourself, lean on the programs and protections available, and take the time to rest and refuel. Stepping away doesn't mean you're abandoning your role, it means you're securing the strength to keep fulfilling it. And when you return, you'll be steadier, stronger, and better equipped to give the care your loved one truly deserves.

Day 283

Stop by a nail salon and ask for a foot or hand massage.
Those ten minutes can seem like heaven.

Sometimes, a quick, affordable indulgence is exactly what your soul needs. You don't have to book a full spa day. Just ten minutes in a quiet chair, having your hands or feet gently massaged, can melt away stress. Let someone care for you for a change. You deserve that kindness. You deserve that stillness. And it might be the reset you didn't know you needed. Don't wait for a special occasion. Don't convince yourself it's too small to matter. Comfort comes in many forms. Let this be one of them.

Day 284

Caregiving is <u>not</u> a thankless job.

It's a myth that caregiving is a thankless job. While it may feel that way in the daily grind, families and friends of your loved one notice and deeply appreciate the care you're giving; even if they don't always say it out loud. Often, gratitude comes in quiet moments or at the very end, when they finally find the words to express what your dedication has meant to them. The truth is, your efforts are seen, felt, and valued more than you realize. Caregiving leaves a lasting imprint of love that speaks louder than any words of thanks could ever convey. The seeds of care you plant now will live on in the stories they tell and the memories they hold. And one day, you may look back and realize that the greatest thank-you was in the connection you both shared.

Day 285

Separate yourself from negative friends and influences.

Caregiving is already hard; you don't need people who make it more complicated. That friend who guilt-trips you? The relative who constantly criticizes but never shows up? Bless and release. Your energy is precious. Surround yourself with people who build you up, not break you down. Choose peace over drama, encouragement over doubt, love over judgment. Letting go of negativity doesn't make you cruel—it makes you wise. This season calls for strength, not extra weight. Create a circle of support that lifts you when you're low and celebrates you when you rise. That's the company you deserve.

Day 286

Define who your safe people will be.

Not everyone can handle your truth... and that's okay. Define your safe people: the ones you can cry with, vent to, and ask for help without judgment or explanation. These are the people who hold space, not opinions. They listen more than they lecture. You don't need many; just one or two will do. Lean on them. Let them be your emergency exits when you need to escape the weight of it all. Safe people make caregiving survivable. They remind you that you're still a person, not just a provider. Identify them early. Keep them close. Let them love you well. And when you forget how strong you are, they'll remind you. Because sometimes the greatest gift in caregiving is knowing you don't have to carry it alone.

Day 287

Realize you may be in a place of constant grieving.

Grief doesn't always come in one big wave; it can come in drips. Caregivers often live in a place of ongoing, unspoken loss: the loss of freedom, routine, health, or who your loved one used to be. This is real grief. And it's okay to name it. You're not "overreacting"; you're mourning things the world doesn't always recognize. Permit yourself to feel it. To cry. To miss what used to be. This isn't weakness; it's humanity. Constant grieving doesn't mean continuous sadness, but it does mean you need regular space to process. Be gentle with yourself. You're carrying a lot.

Day 288

Delegate, delegate, delegate.

You were never meant to do this alone. Delegate like your sanity depends on it—because it does. Let go of the notion that if you don't do it, it won't be done right. You can't carry all the groceries, manage all the meds, and still be a whole, rested human being. Assign tasks—big and small. Trust others with the to-do list and release the guilt. Delegation isn't laziness—it's leadership. You're directing a production, not acting every part. Teach people. Train them if needed. Then let go. You've got more important things to do—like rest, breathe, and just be. Remember, the more you share the load, the longer you can sustain the journey. And in the end, everyone involved feels the gift of contributing to care.

Day 289

You cannot serve from an empty vessel.

Repeat this until it sticks: "I matter, too." Caring for someone else while ignoring your own needs isn't noble, it's unsustainable. Your strength, compassion, and patience are renewable resources, but only if you refill them. Take breaks. Eat well. Get sleep. Say no. Laugh. Move. Breathe. These aren't indulgences, they're maintenance. You're not taking away from your loved one when you care for yourself. You're ensuring that you can continue to show up; not just physically, but fully. You can't pour love from an empty cup. Fill yours regularly. You're worth the time. You're worth the care. And you're better for everyone when you're well.

Day 290

Do not feel guilty about not being able to do it all.

Guilt loves to whisper, "You should be doing more." But here's the truth: no one can do it all. Not you, not anyone. You're not a machine; you're a human with limits. And the fact that you care so much is proof that you're already doing more than most. Let go of the guilt. Embrace the reality. You're doing your best in circumstances that are anything but easy. You don't need to "earn" your rest or justify your boundaries. Repeat after me: "I'm not failing; I'm prioritizing." Give yourself the same grace you offer others. You are enough. Right now. As-is. And on the days when you forget, come back to this truth as many times as you need. Because love, not guilt, is what defines your caregiving.

Day 291

Starting your day with a negative attitude or expectation sets the wrong tone for the entire day.

Mornings set the rhythm. If you wake up already defeated, the whole day feels heavier. Try shifting your mindset before your feet hit the floor. You don't need toxic positivity, just a small, quiet intention. "Today, I'll try again." "Today, I'll give myself grace." Even a single breath of hope can change your direction. It won't fix everything, but it softens the edges. Establish a simple morning ritual that helps you feel grounded. A song. A stretch. A quiet cup of coffee. Don't start in defense mode. Start in care mode. For them and you. Your mindset is your first act of strength each day.

Day 292

Keep a whiteboard in a central spot (or a Google sheet) to capture jobs, due dates, and supplies needed.

Your brain is juggling a lot: appointments, errands, meds, emotions. Give it a break. A central whiteboard or an online Google sheet can serve as the mission control center for your caregiving universe. Jot down tasks, supply needs, upcoming appointments, or even inspirational quotes. Family members can see what's happening and pitch in. No more, "What do you need from the store?" texts... just check the board or sheet. It's a visual brain dump that saves your mental energy for the more emotional parts of caregiving. And when everything's written down in one spot? You get to sleep a little easier.

Day 293

Build a large support team that knows what you don't.

Caregiving is too big for one person to handle alone, and that's why building a strong support team is essential. Surround yourself with people who know what you don't; medical professionals, trusted family members, friends, or local resources, each bringing their expertise and perspective. Maybe that's a nurse who can explain the medical jargon, a friend who's excellent at organizing schedules, or a neighbor who can step in when you need a break. The more voices and skills you have in your corner, the stronger and less overwhelmed you'll feel. You don't have to know everything; you need to know who to call.

Day 294

In-home respite care allows for healthcare aides to provide companionship, nursing services, or both.

If leaving home isn't ideal, in-home respite may be the perfect fit. Trained aides can step in to provide companionship, assist with medications or personal care, and ensure safety while you take a break. Whether you need an afternoon off or a regular schedule, this flexible option gives you breathing room, without your loved one needing to leave their environment. Peace of mind is priceless, and this allows you to rest while knowing someone qualified is holding the space. Ask your doctor, hospice team, or local agency for vetted providers. In-home respite gives your body and soul a chance to reset.

Day 295

Provide step-by-step instructions, illustrated, if possible, for medication and/or medical purposes.

Clear, visual instructions reduce mistakes and ease anxiety, especially for helpers stepping in for the first time. Use simple language and diagrams if needed. "Give one pill at 8 AM with food" is better than "follow the prescription label." Include what to do, when, and how. Add pictures if you can. Laminate it or slip it into a clear folder. When someone else takes over, even briefly, these guides can be the difference between chaos and calm. You're not just delegating, you're empowering others to support you with confidence. And that makes the whole system stronger.

Day 296

Embrace the tiny miracles.

Caregiving is full of long days and short tempers. But tucked in the folds of exhaustion are tiny miracles; fleeting moments that fill your heart in ways words can't. A smile that breaks through confusion. A squeeze of your hand. The quiet stillness of shared presence. These are sacred moments, disguised as ordinary. They won't be in the medical charts, but they'll be etched into your soul. Notice them. Treasure them. Let them be enough when everything else feels too big. In a world that constantly asks for more, these small things whisper. This is what matters most.

Day 297

Employees covered under the Federal Family and Medical Leave Act may be able to take up to 12 weeks of unpaid leave each year to care for relatives.

You may not be aware of it, but the law might be on your side. Under the Family and Medical Leave Act (FMLA), eligible employees can take up to 12 weeks of unpaid, job-protected leave each year to care for an ill family member. That time could be life-changing for both you and them. Talk to your HR department. Understand your rights. Use that time strategically, whether for caregiving, self-care, or recovery. It's not a vacation. It's a necessity. You don't have to push through everything while pretending you're fine. If you qualify, take the leave. Your role at home matters just as much.

Day 298

Laugh at inappropriate things.

Sometimes life is just so ridiculous, all you can do is laugh—and often at the worst possible moments. That's okay. Humor isn't disrespectful; it's human. A well-timed laugh (even if it's dark, awkward, or wildly inappropriate) is often what keeps you from completely unraveling. Caregiving brings absurdity. Laugh at it. With it. Through it. You're not minimizing the hard stuff—you're surviving it. Let laughter break the tension, open the floodgates, or just reset your mood. It's not a sign you're losing it; it's a sign you're coping in your own wonderfully weird way.

Day 299

Build a caregiving village.

Don't just rely on doctors; build your caregiving village. Social workers, care coordinators, therapists, and educators are often the hidden gems of the medical system. They can connect you with services, explain confusing paperwork, and help you advocate for your loved one (and yourself). Ask for referrals. Attend workshops. Find out what programs are available. Medical knowledge is essential, but emotional, logistical, and financial support are equally important. The system is complex, but you're not expected to decipher it on your own. Leverage every helping hand. Support isn't weakness; it's wisdom. And the more informed you are, the more empowered you become.

Day 300

*If you have trouble getting a good night's sleep,
talk to your doctor.*

Sleep deprivation is common, but it's not harmless. It impacts your mood, memory, patience, and immune system. If you're tossing, turning, or waking up more tired than rested, speak up. Don't just power through. Discuss with your doctor strategies such as sleep hygiene, melatonin, routines, or other support options. Sometimes a medical issue (anxiety, pain, or medication side effects) interferes. You deserve real rest. Not just naps between tasks, but deep, restorative sleep. Caregiving is demanding, and you need a solid foundation to keep going.

Day 301

Even in your darkest days, you do an important job, whether anyone realizes it or not.

You may not hear it. You may not feel it. But what you do matters. Deeply. Your acts of care are changing someone's world, even when appreciation feels scarce. Know that you are seen. You are valued and loved. The exhaustion, the doubt, the invisible weight; you're carrying it all with strength that goes far beyond words. Please don't wait for applause to believe in your impact. You are doing important work. And just because the world isn't cheering doesn't mean your love isn't recognized. In the quiet, in the chaos, you are making a difference. And you are not alone.

Day 302

Secure resources before making changes to your home.

Before making any changes to your home for caregiving, such as adding a ramp, renovating a bathroom, or creating a more accessible bedroom, take the time to research and secure available resources first. There are programs, grants, and local agencies that can help cover or offset the cost of these modifications, but here's the catch: once the work is started, those funds or resources are often no longer available. Do your homework up front, talk to local organizations like the Office for the Aging or community nonprofits, and see what assistance you qualify for. A little planning can save you a lot of money and stress down the road.

Day 303

Resource: eldercare.gov

This site connects you directly with services in your local area through the Eldercare Locator. You plug in your zip code, and suddenly you're holding a map of nearby aging-related support: transportation, meals, legal help, and more. Run by the U.S. Administration on Aging, this tool helps you find real people to talk to, not just webpages. Need to know where your mom can get adult day care or how to apply for a local aid program? Start here. It's a calm port in the storm of information overload. No guesswork, just guidance.

Day 304

Find your tribe.

When the road gets long, you need people who walk with you, not just cheer from the sidelines. A church, spiritual group, or values-aligned community can provide emotional support, meals, rides, prayers, hugs, and a sense of presence. Sometimes, they'll just sit beside your silence, and that's the kind of tribe you want. Seek out those who see caregiving not as a burden, but as a sacred service. Let them hold you up when you're tired. Let them remind you you're not invisible. Whether it's a faith-based community or a group that cares, find your people, and let them love you forward. Community doesn't erase the hard, but it makes it bearable. And in their care, you'll find strength you didn't know you had.

Day 305

Getting help allows you to spend time with the person you're caring for in a better, more personal way.

You didn't sign up to manage medications and paperwork—you signed up because you love them. But the tasks can crowd out the relationship. Accepting help with chores, errands, or routines gives you something priceless: time. Help isn't just about lightening the load; it's about making room for connection. You get to be less of a taskmaster and more of a companion. You get to look them in the eye instead of racing the clock. And that's the kind of caregiving that nourishes both of you. Less doing. More being. Let helpers make that possible.

Day 306

Look in the mirror and say, "Good job!"

It might feel silly but do it anyway. Look yourself in the eyes and say, "You're doing a great job." Because you are. Even when no one's clapping, even when no one notices, you notice. You know what you've endured, accomplished, and navigated. Give yourself credit for every small win, because they add up. You are worthy of encouragement from the inside out. And if today was messy? If you forgot something or lost your patience? Hug yourself anyway. You're showing up, and that counts more than perfection ever could. You are your own most prominent advocate. Don't wait for praise to be given to you; give it to yourself freely.

Day 307

Have a basket full of forgiveness for yourself as you are learning, and for your loved one.

You'll make mistakes. They'll make mistakes. That's not failure, it's humanity. Keep a basket of forgiveness close. Pull from it often. For the moment, you lost your temper. For a time, they refused help again. For the forgotten appointments, the harsh words, or the guilt you carry, forgive yourself and forgive them. This road is hard, and everyone's doing the best they can in bodies and hearts that sometimes betray them. Forgiveness won't erase the hard, but it will soften it. Let go of the blame. Lean into love. And remember, grace isn't just something you give, it's something you deserve.

Day 308

Have conversations with aging parents and family members while they are still healthy and of sound mind.

Don't wait for a crisis to start talking. When aging parents are still healthy and sharp, that's your window. Discuss healthcare wishes, living arrangements, finances, and what matters most to them. It might feel awkward at first, but these conversations bring clarity and reduce confusion in the long run. Make it part of everyday conversation, maybe over coffee, not during a hospital stay. It's not morbid; it's responsible. And it's kind. You're not just preparing; you're honoring their voice. You'll thank yourself in the future. So will they. Start small, but start soon. These talks are a gift. Give it while everyone can still give back.

Day 309

Make sure to tell your doctor that you're a caregiver.

You're not just a caregiver; you're also a patient. And your health matters, too. Let your doctor know what your caregiving life looks like: the hours, the stress, the demands. It gives them context for your sleep patterns, blood pressure, mental health, and energy levels. Be honest about your concerns, both physical and emotional. You might be powering through, but don't mask burnout with a smile. Your provider can only support what they know. So, speak up and ask questions. Advocate for yourself with the same fire you use for your loved one. You're a priority, too.

Day 310

Help prepare a list of key questions for medical and dental visits.

Doctor visits can be overwhelming, especially when you're trying to remember every detail. Help your loved one create a list of key questions in advance, including changes in symptoms, side effects, medications, and potential 'what-if' scenarios. Write it down. Bring it along. This empowers them to stay engaged and ensures nothing important gets lost in the moment. Please encourage them to speak up because it's their care, after all. And if they feel shy? You can help advocate. A prepared visit is a more productive one. Questions aren't bothersome; they're the key to better outcomes. So, prep the list, bring a pen, and don't be afraid to ask.

Day 311

Recognize that often caregiving is not a choice.

Caregiving is often not a choice; it can happen suddenly, leaving both you and your loved one facing a new reality you never planned for. While you're adjusting to the demands of care, they're coping with the profound loss of independence and control. And here's the tricky part: you won't adjust at the same pace. One of you may find acceptance or a new rhythm faster, while the other struggles to catch up emotionally or mentally. That's normal. Give each other space and grace to move through the process. Start with simple routines, seek support where you can, and remember that this is a journey you're learning to navigate together, even if you're not always in step.

Day 312

Greatness is measured in tenderness and compassion.

A truly generous heart notices, softens, and shows up. Caregiving is the purest expression of this kind of greatness. It's not flashy, but it is fierce. To offer your time, energy, and love is a quiet, sacred strength, even when no one is watching. So, if you ever doubt your worth, remember this: the compassionate way you care is your greatest strength. You are living out the highest version of what it means to be human. That's something to be deeply proud of. Your love is creating a legacy far greater than any accolade or achievement. And long after the tasks are forgotten, the impact of your care will remain.

Day 313

*In the heart of every caregiver is a knowing that
you are all connected.*

Caregiving reveals the beautiful truth that we're not meant to go through life alone. In helping someone else, we discover parts of ourselves, such as patience, empathy, and tenderness that we didn't know we had. And in every act of care, we're reminded: we are all bound together. Today, it's you helping them; someday, someone may help you. What you give flows beyond you. It shapes families, generations, and even how you see yourself. Care is never wasted. It lives on. You're not just giving your time; you're building a bridge between hearts.

Day 314

*You will never realize how strong you are until being
strong is the only choice you have.*

There's a kind of strength that doesn't shout; it simply shows up. It's the strength that carries you forward when everything feels impossible, yet you keep going anyway. It's crying in the shower, then finding a way to smile later. It's staying, serving, and loving through the mess. You didn't choose this road, but you are rising to it in ways you may not even see. You're not weak for feeling overwhelmed; you're strong because you refuse to quit. Strength isn't the absence of fear or fatigue; it's the courage to keep moving through them. You may not always feel heroic, but trust me, you are. Every small act of care is evidence of a resilience that grows stronger with each step. And one day, you'll look back and realize you carried far more than you thought possible.

Day 315

Get through today, but an understanding of what's coming next can help you prepare and reduce stress.

Yes, some days are pure survival mode, but don't forget to zoom out every so often. Understanding what's ahead (even just a little) can give you time to plan, delegate, or emotionally brace yourself. Talk to care providers about what's likely to change. Ask other caregivers about the next chapter. Keep notes. Being proactive doesn't mean you're trying to control everything; it means you're making space to breathe. Even a rough sketch of what's coming can help you feel less caught off guard. Today is important, but so is being ready for tomorrow. You're not just surviving, you're building resilience.

Day 316

No one is a "perfect" caregiver.

Guilt may come with the caregiver package, but perfection doesn't. You'll forget things. You'll lose your temper. You'll wish for a break. None of that makes you a bad caregiver; it makes you human. There's no medal for doing it all flawlessly, and there shouldn't be. What matters most is that you keep showing up with love, even when it's messy. Forgive yourself for the moments you wish had gone differently. Learn, grow, and keep moving forward. You're doing an incredibly hard job with courage and heart, and that is more than enough. Your loved one doesn't need perfection; they need you, present and real. And someday, you'll see that your imperfect love was exactly what made it powerful.

Day 317

Remove throw rugs, they are an immense trip hazard.

They may look cozy, but throw rugs are one of the biggest hidden safety risks in a caregiving environment. One wrong step can lead to a fall, an injury, or something even more serious. For those with mobility challenges, vision changes, or shuffling gaits, rugs can be like banana peels in disguise. Be proactive and don't wait until after an accident. Remove them altogether or secure them firmly with non-slip backing and rug tape. Check every walkway, especially in high-risk areas like the bathroom, kitchen, and bedroom. A fall prevention plan doesn't begin after a fall; it begins today. A simple change now can save you from a world of complications later. Safety always comes before style. Protecting your loved one's steps protects their independence. And when you create a safer home, you also create more peace of mind for yourself.

Day 318

When someone asks if they can help, pull out your to-do list and dole out tasks.

Keep a living list of errands, needs, and small tasks, such as picking up prescriptions, mowing the lawn, bringing dinner, or sitting for an hour. Write it down as it comes up. The next time someone says, "Let me know what I can do," you won't be scrambling for an answer; you'll be ready. When help is offered, you've got options. You don't have to do it all. And you don't have to pretend you're fine when you're not. Delegate without guilt because people want to help. Make it easy for them to step in. Your list is a lifeline.

Day 319

While you are taking on new and additional responsibilities, you are still allowed a life of your own.

Caregiving may fill your calendar, but it should never erase your identity. You are still a person with passions, dreams, and needs. You're allowed to laugh. To rest, see friends, and even read a book with zero educational value. Choosing joy doesn't mean you're abandoning your loved one, it means you're preserving the energy to keep showing up for them. Your life doesn't end because theirs has changed. Carve out space for yourself, even if it's small. You matter, not just as a caregiver, but as a whole, beautiful, complete human being. And the more you honor your own life, the more fully you can honor theirs.

Day 320

Some assisted living homes and memory care facilities accept people needing short-term care.

Need a break longer than a day or two? Traveling for a wedding or just needing time to reset? Many facilities offer short-term stays where your loved one receives full-time care, meals, and supervision. This type of respite can be a game-changer. It's okay to need time away. It's OK not to feel guilty about it. You're not abandoning your loved one, you're trusting professionals so you can return rested, recharged, and more present. Visit the facility beforehand, ask about daily routines, and share your loved one's preferences. A break this big might feel scary, but it can also be deeply restorative.

Day 321

Kindness comes back in unexpected ways.

Kindness has a way of circling back to you, often when you need it most. A smile or a thank-you to the nurses, receptionists, pharmacists, or aides who cross your path can go further than you realize. That extra bit of gratitude might mean a nurse goes out of their way to check in on your loved one, a receptionist squeezes you into a premium appointment slot, or a pharmacist finds a coupon or discount on a pricey medication. It's not about expecting favors—it's about building relationships and goodwill with the people who are part of your care team. In the world of caregiving, a little kindness can open unexpected doors.

Day 322

Learn how to communicate with doctors effectively.

Doctors are experts, but you're the expert on your loved one. Don't be intimidated. Ask questions. Repeat back what you've heard to ensure you understand. Bring a notebook or voice recorder. Write down symptoms and side effects ahead of time. If something doesn't feel right, say so. You are your loved one's advocate. You don't need a medical degree to ask, "Can you explain that again?" or "Is there another option?" Clarity leads to better care. Don't rush out of the room if you are still confused. Speak up. You belong in that conversation. You have a right to know and to be heard. And remember, when you speak with confidence, you not only protect your loved one, but you also empower yourself.

Day 323

Take time to do what makes your soul happy.

Your calendar may be packed, but your soul still deserves space. Joy isn't selfish, it's medicine. Whether it's dancing in the kitchen, gardening, painting, journaling, or watching your favorite guilty-pleasure show, carve out moments that make you feel yourself. Even 15 minutes can restore your spirit. This isn't an "extra" on your to-do list—it's vital maintenance. When your soul is nourished, your care becomes more peaceful and powerful. So go ahead, laugh out loud, take that detour, play that song again. You deserve joy, not just survival.

Day 324

Everyone has unique challenges.

It's easy to assume others have it easier, but most people are carrying burdens you can't see. Another caregiver. Another loss. Another quiet heartbreak. Lead with compassion, not comparison. When your heart stretches instead of hardens, you make space for grace. And that grace? It always finds its way back to you. Even when you feel invisible, remember you're not walking this road alone; you're one of many moving forward with courage. Kindness may not fix everything, but it softens the sharp edges of the journey for you and those beside you. Everyone is fighting a battle, whether seen or unseen. Gentleness costs nothing, yet it can mean everything. And when we choose to walk softly together, the load becomes lighter for us all.

Day 325

Get creative when planting seeds of change.

Sometimes the best way to encourage change is to get creative with how you plant the seed. Your loved one might resist a suggestion coming directly from you, especially if it feels like you're "telling them what to do." But when the same idea comes from someone else, like a trusted friend, a doctor, or even through a casual conversation with another family member, it can be received with far less resistance. The goal isn't to push, but to guide gently, creating opportunities for them to feel ownership over the decision. A well-placed word from the right voice can make all the difference.

Day 326

There will always be an urgency to life when
you are a caregiver.

When you're a caregiver, life often feels like it's lived on high alert. There's always something pressing: medications to give, appointments to schedule, meals to prepare, or unexpected needs that pop up without warning. That constant sense of urgency can leave you feeling like you can never truly rest. While you can't eliminate the demands, you *can* create small moments of calm; whether that's pausing for a deep breath, stepping outside for a few minutes, or planning quiet breaks into your day. Accept that the urgency will always be there, but don't let it rob you of every moment of peace. You need both to endure.

Day 327

Love yourself; you are worthy.

You don't have to earn your worth through service or self-sacrifice. You are worthy right now—before the to-do list is done, before the gratitude is spoken, before the mess is cleaned. Look in the mirror and say it: "I am enough." Love the version of yourself that's tired, unshowered, emotional, and showing up anyway. Caregiving doesn't strip away your value; it reveals it. You are not "just" anything. You are a powerful, vital, beautiful human. Don't wait for someone else to remind you. Say it now. Say it often. Because the love you give to others? You deserve it, too.

Day 328

Rotate the tasks on your care calendar so no one gets burned out on a single task.

Even the most willing helpers can burn out when they're stuck in a repetitive cycle. Avoid the "Mom always cooks" or "Bob always drives" pattern by rotating tasks. Create a shared calendar with grocery runs, medication pickups, or visits, and mix it up. Let everyone carry a little, instead of a few carrying a lot. It's better for you, better for them, and better for your loved one. A rotating rhythm fosters shared responsibility and helps prevent resentment. You're building a team here, not a hierarchy. Keep it simple. Keep it fair. Keep it moving.

Day 329

Read: Finding God in the Storms of Life by Bill Hybels

When caregiving shakes your faith or raises more questions than answers, this book steps in like a steady hand. Bill Hybels doesn't minimize pain; he acknowledges it. Through spiritual reflection, he reminds you that God is not absent in the storm but right there with you in the eye of it. If you're looking for strength, comfort, or a reminder that your heart matters to God, this book offers that gently. Faith doesn't erase the hard; it walks you through it. This one helps you hold on.

Day 330

Some people might assume caregiving for a spouse is easy... it's not.

Some people assume that caregiving for a spouse must be easier because you already know them so well, but that couldn't be further from the truth. In many ways, it's harder. The dynamic of your relationship shifts, and the person who was once your equal partner may now depend on you for almost everything. That shift can stir up grief, frustration, and exhaustion, right alongside the love and loyalty that keep you moving forward. It's okay to admit that it's not easy. Loving someone deeply doesn't make the physical, emotional, and mental weight of caregiving any lighter, but it does give you a powerful reason to keep showing up. This role asks you to carry both partner and caregiver at once. It is a balancing act no one prepares you for, yet through the hardest days, your love is what transforms duty into devotion.

Day 331

If you have a child with special needs, ensure that life is not all about them. Your other children need to know they are special too... in a different way.

It's easy to pour all your energy into the child who needs the most, but don't let your other children feel invisible. They may not say it, but they notice when everything revolves around their sibling. Make time for their stories, their victories, and their weird jokes. Celebrate them, too. You don't have to split yourself evenly—just intentionally. Even a 10-minute "just us" moment makes a difference. Remind them they're seen, loved, and unique, not just "the sibling of..." You're not ignoring your caregiving role; you're expanding your love in both directions. All your children deserve to feel chosen in your presence.

Day 332

Many communities have classes specifically about the disease your loved one is facing.

Knowledge is power, especially when caregiving feels overwhelming. Community classes can offer more than just information; they offer connection. Whether in person or online, these programs explain the disease process, care techniques, and resources that can help alleviate your burden. You'll hear from professionals and other caregivers, and suddenly, you won't feel so alone. These classes may be offered through local hospitals, senior centers, nonprofits, or disease-specific organizations. Don't assume you have to figure everything out alone. Others have walked this path and have left wisdom behind. Learn, listen, and go get the tools you deserve.

Day 333

---

*Meet other caregivers to alleviate isolation,
share stories and ideas.*

Caregiving can be lonely, but it doesn't have to be. Connecting with others who "get it" can be a lifeline. No need to explain the exhaustion, the guilt, or why you cried over spilled soup; they already know. Join a local group or find one online. Share your story and swap tips. Ask questions. Or sit in the comfort of people who understand. You'll gain new insights, practical help, and maybe even a friend. Sometimes the best medicine isn't advice; it's "me too." Caregiving is heavy, but it's lighter when carried together.

Day 334

---

*What you're doing, even the little, monotonous tasks,
is making a difference.*

Filling pillboxes. Making meals. Repeating the same story. Wiping down counters. Scheduling appointments. These tasks may seem invisible, but they create comfort, stability, and dignity for someone who needs it. They matter. You matter. Love doesn't always roar. Sometimes it's quiet. Repetitive. Undramatic. And still, it's everything. Don't underestimate the sacredness of the mundane. You are building a legacy of love, one routine at a time. So, the next time you feel like you're doing "nothing special," remember: the daily grind is the gold. And your care is a quiet miracle in motion.

Day 335

Prioritize, make lists, and establish a daily routine.

Routines create calm in the chaos. When everything feels unpredictable, having a list or rhythm gives you a sense of control. Prioritize what matters most. Let go of the nonessentials; yes, even that elaborate Thanksgiving dinner you used to host. Say no to requests that sap your strength and yes to what brings peace. Lists help your brain rest. Routines help your day flow. And boundaries? They protect your sanity. Simplify where you can. Outsource what you must. You're not failing, you're adapting. That's wisdom. And wisdom is what gets you through.

Day 336

Never forget to look after #1... yourself.

It may feel selfish, but it's a strategic move. If you neglect your care, your ability to care for someone else will eventually unravel. Prioritize sleep, meals, movement, connection, whatever keeps you functioning. Don't wait until you're running on fumes to check in with yourself. Treat your well-being like it's non-negotiable, because it is. You're not just a caregiver—you're a whole person with your own needs. Put yourself on the list. Not last. Not "if there's time." Now. You're your first patient. Care for yourself accordingly.

Day 337

If you have trouble getting a good night's sleep,
talk to your doctor.

Sleep is not a luxury; it's a lifeline. Without it, your body can't heal, your mind can't reset, and your patience wears thin. If you've been running on fumes for too long, it's time to stop treating exhaustion like a badge of honor. Talk to your doctor. Explore options. Sometimes the fix is routine-based; sometimes it's more profound. Whatever the cause, please don't ignore it. Sleep affects everything from immunity to mood to memory. Prioritize rest like it's medication. You're caring for someone else, but you're still responsible for your own well-being. Start with sleep. Everything gets clearer from there.

Day 338

Offering care means being a companion, not a superior.

Caregiving is not about control; it's about connection. You're not "in charge" of someone; you're walking alongside them in one of life's toughest chapters. Listen more than you speak. Include rather than dictate. Respect their wishes, their pace, and their voice, even when they can't always express it. This isn't a hierarchy; it's a relationship. One grounded in dignity. Remember: your role isn't to lead the journey, it's to hold a steady hand on the path. Companion over commander, always. That mindset shift makes all the difference for them and you.

Day 339

*People will say stupid things often from
a place of ignorance.*

"Oh wow, I could never do what you do." "At least they're still alive." "Maybe you're overreacting." Yep. People mean well... but wow, do they miss the mark. Their words might sting, but usually, they come from not knowing what to say. Take a breath. You don't have to educate everyone. And you don't have to absorb their ignorance as truth. Vent to someone safe, laugh if you can, and keep it moving. You're doing something most people can't even imagine. Let their words roll off your shoulders. Save your energy for those who understand.

Day 340

*Create and share a list of essential telephone numbers,
including emergency contacts, local pharmacies,
and medical providers.*

In an emergency, you don't want to be fumbling through your phone or trying to read tiny print with shaky hands. Create a clear, easy-to-read list of all essential contacts, such as doctors, specialists, local hospitals, pharmacies, family, neighbors, and poison control. Print a bold copy to post by the front door or on the fridge. Tuck another into your bag or glove compartment. And don't forget to share a digital version, such as a Google sheet, with any backup caregivers, so it's always accessible, even from a mobile device. For loved ones or helpers with vision challenges, large print isn't just helpful, it's lifesaving. It's a simple step that delivers tremendous peace of mind when every second counts.

Day 341

*Be open to new technologies that can help you
care for your loved one.*

Tech isn't just for teenagers and spreadsheets; it's a lifeline for caregivers. From medication reminders and smart home tools to medical apps and digital support groups, technology can ease your load in practical ways. Please don't dismiss it because it's unfamiliar. Explore it. Ask others what's helped them. Watch a tutorial. You might find something that gives you back time, energy, or peace of mind. You don't have to be tech-savvy; just tech-curious. There are tools available that can help reduce stress, improve safety, and keep you organized. Use what works. Let tech be your assistant, not another burden. You've earned every shortcut. And remember, every minute saved on tasks is a minute you can give back to yourself, or to the moments that matter most.

Day 342

Do not underestimate the power of routine.

Routines can feel silly, tedious, or even unnecessary to you, but for your loved one, they can be a lifeline. That predictable rhythm— whether it's a favorite morning show, a certain snack at the same time each day, or a nightly wind-down can bring a deep sense of comfort and security. For someone whose world may feel unpredictable or overwhelming, these small rituals are anchors that reduce stress and confusion. Even if it seems trivial, remember that what feels repetitive to you might be the very thing that makes your loved one feel safe, seen, and steady.

Day 343

*Some care centers provide care for both older
adults and young children.*

Respite care doesn't just give you a break; it offers stimulation, routine, and companionship for your loved one, too. Some adult day programs even pair elders with children for shared activities, creating joyful, intergenerational moments that benefit both groups. These programs often include meals, light exercise, crafts, or music. You might be surprised how much peace you feel knowing your loved one is engaged and cared for while you rest, run errands, or simply breathe. Respite isn't selfish; it's sustainability. Explore local centers. Even a few hours can make a world of difference—for both of you.

Day 344

Set realistic goals.

Rome wasn't built in a day, and neither is a caregiver's to-do list. Big tasks can feel paralyzing. So, break them down: one phone call, one form, one drawer at a time. Progress is progress, even when it's small. Celebrate the little wins. Write them down. Check them off. You're not lazy, you're human. Life isn't a sprint; it's a series of tiny, purposeful steps. When you zoom out, you'll see that every small task brought you closer to stability. Don't let overwhelm steal your momentum. Take the next small step. That's enough for today.

Day 345

Watch out for signs of overwhelm.

Pay attention to the subtle signs that you're reaching your limit: feelings of overwhelm, constant worry, irritability, or losing interest in things you once enjoyed. Emotional signals like sadness or hopelessness can creep in, and physical symptoms like frequent headaches or fatigue are often your body's way of waving a red flag. Some caregivers even find themselves leaning on unhealthy coping habits, like increased alcohol use, without realizing it. These signs don't mean you're weak; they tell you're human and in need of care, too. When you notice these patterns, pause, ask for help, and make time to reset before burnout takes over.

Day 346

Tend to your emotional garden daily.

Resentment starts quietly. A sigh. A skipped break. A "Why do I always...?" left unanswered. Left unchecked, it takes root. Grows bitterness. Chokes joy. That's why emotional weeding matters. Tend to your inner world. Check in with yourself daily. Journal. Talk. Rest. Ask for help. Say no when needed. Say yes to yourself, too. Like a garden, your heart needs watering, care, light, and breathing room. Don't let resentment take over your soil. You're not meant to give endlessly without care. You're allowed to grow peace alongside purpose.

Day 347

*Some days you need to take it day by day,
hour by hour, or minute by minute.*

When everything feels overwhelming, zoom in. You don't have to solve tomorrow today. Just breathe through this hour. Then the next. Sometimes, survival mode is sacred. One moment, one task, one deep breath at a time. The good news? No feeling lasts forever. Not this frustration. Not this fatigue. Not this chaos. Tomorrow might offer a little more ease. But today? Just focus on what's right in front of you. That's not weakness—it's wisdom. Some days, all you can do is keep going. And that's enough.

Day 348

*Take a deep breath and give yourself credit for
your caring nature.*

Take a deep breath and really hear this: you are doing meaningful, life-changing work. It may not come with applause or medals, but the impact is real. The love you give, such as sacrifices, patience, and steady presence, shapes someone's world in ways that matter. Even when it goes unnoticed, it still counts. Give yourself credit for showing up, loving fully, and for trying again on the hard days. There is strength in your quiet courage. The difference you're making will ripple far beyond what you can see. Trust that truth and let it steady you when the weight feels heavy. And, never forget: the way you show up in ordinary moments is extraordinary to someone else.

Day 349

*Take comfort in knowing that you don't need to
fill the silence to make a visit meaningful.*

Silence isn't awkward. It's sacred, especially in caregiving, where presence often speaks louder than words. Don't pressure yourself to entertain, explain, or fix every moment. Just being there is powerful. Holding a hand. Sitting quietly. Breathing in rhythm. These are acts of love. Your calmness is a gift. Your stillness is enough. Some of the most meaningful moments don't require conversation; they need compassion. So, settle into the silence. Let it comfort, connect, and heal. You're doing beautifully, even when no words are spoken.

Day 350

Let go of what you cannot control.

So much of caregiving is beyond your control: disease progression, family dynamics, schedules, and the reactions of others. Trying to manage it all will only leave you frustrated, exhausted, and drained. The key is to shift your focus to what is in your power: how you show up, how you respond, when you rest, and what you ask for. Letting go doesn't mean giving up; it means protecting your peace. Surrendering the unchangeable frees you to give your best energy to the things you can influence. It's not about doing everything, it's about doing the right things with the strength you have. This shift takes practice, but over time it becomes a daily act of resilience that lightens your load and steadies your spirit. And in that steadiness, you'll find room for hope, patience, and even moments of joy.

Day 351

Caregiving will touch everyone at some point in their life.

Caregiving is universal; it touches every life eventually. You're part of a global circle of empathy and love. This isn't a solo act; it's a shared story. Some people understand because they've walked it. Others will know when they do. You're not alone. You're part of something deeply human and profoundly noble. When you feel invisible, remember that what you're doing echoes across generations. And one day, someone may look at you and say, "Because of you, I know how to love like that." Keep going. You're part of something bigger than you know.

Day 352

Continue to check in with a care facility, even after the honeymoon period has passed.

Even if your first tours and visits to a care facility were impressive, don't assume that level of care will always stay the same. There's often a honeymoon period where everything feels perfect, but over time, routines can shift, staff can change, and details can slip through the cracks. Keep checking in regularly, not just on scheduled visits. Drop by unexpectedly when you can, observe how your loved one is being treated, and talk to other residents or families. Staying vigilant isn't about being distrustful; it's about ensuring your loved one continues to receive the care, respect, and attention they deserve.

Day 353

Try to achieve a better balance in your life... just don't expect those around you to like it.

When you start setting boundaries and saying no to burnout, not everyone will clap. Some folks are comfortable with your over-functioning. But your job isn't to keep others comfortable, it's to keep yourself healthy. Balance might mean disappointing someone. It might mean opting out of things you used to handle. And yes, it might get awkward. But don't let guilt talk louder than your body or soul. You're not being selfish. You're smart. Balance doesn't mean equality; it means sustainability. You can't serve well from the edge of collapse.

Day 354

Patience is the #1 resource needed for caregiving.

Patience is the single most valuable resource in caregiving, and it's tested daily. Even if you consider yourself a patient person, you may find certain people or situations that push every button you have. That doesn't make you a bad caregiver; it makes you human. But when your patience starts running on fumes, it's a signal that something needs to shift; whether that means taking a break, asking for help, or rethinking how you approach a task. Recognize that limit isn't weakness; it's wisdom. Replenish your patience, and you'll show up with the compassion and steadiness your loved one truly needs.

Day 355

Say No to requests that are draining.

Your energy is not unlimited. Every "yes" you give to someone else is a "no" to something else; often your own rest, peace, or priorities. You're not required to be available to everyone all the time. Begin to say no to things that deplete you. Kindly. Clearly. Firmly. Protect your time like the resource it is. You don't need an excuse. "No" is a complete sentence. Saying no doesn't make you unkind; it makes you sustainable. Create space for rest, creativity, connection, and joy. Say no to the draining so you can say yes to what matters. You are worth it.

Day 356

Caregiving takes strength of mind, heart, and body.

Caregiving demands strength; not just emotionally, but physically, too. Lifting, transferring, and supporting your loved one can take a real toll on your body if you're not prepared. Building functional strength through simple exercises, along with regular stretching or yoga, can make a big difference in preventing pulled muscles and injuries. Your mind and heart also need that same attention because staying grounded, resilient, and compassionate takes energy. Think of your body, mind, and heart as a team; caring for all three isn't optional, it's essential. The stronger you are in every sense, the better you can care for someone else.

Day 357

Choose and share a safe word with those closest to you so they know when you are reaching a breaking point and need help... now!

You shouldn't have to explain when you're at your edge. That's why having a safe word with your close support circle can be a game-changer. It's a no-questions-asked signal: "I'm maxed out. I need a break. I need backup." Choose something memorable, even humorous, if that fits your vibe: "pineapple" or "unicorn" works just fine. The point is clarity. You're not being dramatic, you're being proactive. When words are hard, let one word do the work. Give your people the cue to show up because burnout doesn't need to arrive before support does.

Day 358

Be prepared to do things you never thought you'd have to do.

Caregiving rewrites the script on what you thought you'd be doing in life. You'll become a part-time nurse, emotional anchor, negotiator, meal-prepper, and late-night Googler of symptoms you can't pronounce. It's strange, sacred work. Be prepared to surprise yourself. To rise when you thought you'd fall. To love through things you didn't think you could handle. It won't always be graceful, but it will be growth. You may feel like you're winging it (and you are), but somehow, you'll keep showing up. That's not just bravery. That's transformation. Let it change you, and honor every version of you along the way.

Day 359

Stay vigilant for signs of bitterness and resentment. Those feelings should be warning signs that you need to support yourself.

Bitterness isn't bad, it's a message. A red flag waving from your emotional dashboard saying, "Hey… something's off." Please don't ignore it. Bitterness often stems from feelings of depletion, unspoken needs, or unshared burdens. It doesn't mean you don't love the person you're caring for, it means you're running dry. Before it spills into your relationships, let it signal a shift: It's time to rest, reset, and receive. Don't wait until you explode. You're not a robot. You're a human with limits. And when you take care of those limits, you create room for peace to grow again.

Day 360

Meditating or simply sitting in silence for five or ten minutes a day can make all the difference.

Taking just five or ten minutes a day to sit quietly or meditate can make a huge difference in how you feel. Your body will often tell you how stressed you are, through tight shoulders, a racing mind, or exhaustion, so take that as a cue to pause and listen. If you're new to meditating, start simple: focus on your breath or try an app like *Calm* to guide you. Those few minutes of stillness can reset your mind, relax your body, and give you the clarity and strength to handle the next challenge with more ease.

Day 361

While the loss is permanent, the season for mourning is not.

Grief arrives like a storm, but it doesn't stay forever. It changes form—softens, deepens, even surprises you. The loss may always ache, but mourning will evolve. There will come a day when you laugh without guilt, and when the memory brings more warmth than tears. Permit yourself to heal at your own pace. There is no timeline. No "right way." But know this: you are allowed to move forward while still holding love. Mourning is a season, not a sentence. And joy is not betrayal, it's a beautiful part of remembering well.

Day 362

Send your care calendar to family, friends, and supporters a month in advance.

Planning gives people time to actually show up. A care calendar isn't just for organization; it's an invitation. By sharing it early, you allow your support circle to carve out time and provide real help. Whether it's meal delivery, errands, or companionship shifts, giving them notice removes the stress from both sides. It turns vague offers of "Let me know if you need anything" into actual action. Make it easy for others to help. A little planning now brings a lot of peace later. Don't just manage the calendar... share it.

Day 363

*While you can excel in some areas, perfection
isn't required or expected.*

Perfection is a myth, and an exhausting one at that. You're not being measured by how flawless your caregiving is. You're being measured by your presence, your effort, and your love. That's what counts. You may forget a detail, lose your patience, or drop a ball. Welcome to humanity. None of that negates the beauty of your heart. You're doing incredible things under incredible pressure. Stop holding yourself to an impossible standard. Your loved one doesn't need a perfect caregiver; they need you. And you, dear one, are doing great.

Day 364

You must take time to do things you enjoy.

Yes, there is joy in caregiving, but you also deserve joy that is just yours. A favorite book. A hobby. Music, nature, movement, art. These aren't luxuries, they're lifelines. If you've forgotten what makes you feel alive, it's time to remember. You are still allowed to delight in something, to laugh, to be light-hearted, even in a heavy season. You're not abandoning your loved one; you're preserving your spirit so you can show up well. Care for yourself like someone who matters because you do. Immensely. Your happiness doesn't subtract from your caregiving; it fuels it. In protecting your own joy, you give your loved one permission to hold on to theirs, too.

Day 365

*Sometimes the most helpful thing you can
do is not jump in.*

As a caregiver, it's natural to want to ease every struggle, prevent every stumble, and smooth every rough edge. But sometimes, helping means stepping back. Let your loved one try; even if it takes longer, even if it's imperfect. Preserving independence, even in small ways, can restore a sense of dignity and control. It's not about doing less; it's about doing thoughtfully. Ask, "Do they *need* help, or do I *need* to help?" That pause can be powerful. Support doesn't always mean solving; it can mean witnessing, encouraging, and honoring their effort without interruption.

What's Next?

This book closes here, but the wisdom within it will stay with you. Every page has been a gift from caregivers who've traveled the road before you, offering their stories so your steps may feel a little lighter.

As you've journeyed through the pages, you've discovered the profound truth expressed in the quote:

"Wisdom is the reward of experience and should be shared."

Let the lessons shared in this book inspire you to move forward with purpose. Your experiences and lessons are your unique wisdom—valuable treasures meant to be shared. Each of us has the power to uplift and inspire others. Let's keep learning from each other, growing together, and spreading positivity and wisdom wherever life takes us.

Finally, please take a moment to scan below and leave a review on Amazon. I read each one, and your feedback helps shape the future of the Wisdom & Warnings series.

About the Author

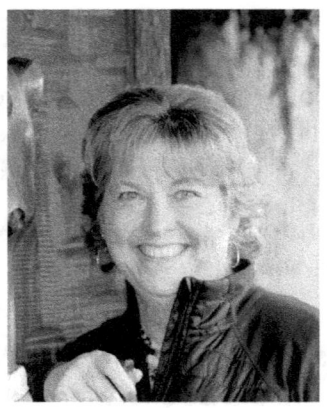

Jen Fort is a writer, speaker, coach, and reinvention catalyst who believes shared wisdom helps people feel less alone and more capable of moving forward. As the creator of the *Wisdom & Warnings* series, Jen gathers insight from real people navigating life's biggest transitions and passes it along with heart, honesty, and encouragement. Her work is rooted in a simple truth: clarity often comes *after* action, and no one is meant to figure out life's hard moments alone. Through her books, talks, and conversations, Jen helps people move forward messy, brave, and more confident than they felt before.

Visit www.iamjenfort.com to:

- Share a lesson or hard-earned insight, and possibly have your wisdom included in a future *Wisdom & Warnings* book.
- Access free resources and tools designed to support people navigating life transitions.
- Be the first to know about new *Wisdom & Warnings* releases, projects, and special offerings.
- Learn how Jen supports groups through speaking, workshops, and coaching focused on reinvention, connection, and real-life wisdom.